T0173658

About the Author

Registered Nutritionist Jenna Hope is passionate and dedicated to optimising people's health and wellbeing. Jenna's interest in nutrition stems from her enthusiasm towards food from a young age. Aged sixteen, she changed her high-sugar, low-fibre diet for one richer in whole foods and noticed the benefits to her energy levels, skin health and mental wellbeing. Consequently, Jenna became fascinated by the way in which food could affect us, and went on to spend five years at university studying nutrition.

Now with an undergraduate degree and a masters in Human Nutrition, and extensive experience in the field, Jenna has a deep appreciation for the complex relationship between food and physiology. Using an evidence-based, non-judgemental and practical approach, Jenna works closely with individuals, brands and large companies to help them implement smarter strategies for nutrition and to support health and wellbeing for the long term. It is her mission to inspire and educate individuals on the smart ways nutrition can enhance your life.

Jenna is considered an expert voice within the media and is regularly called upon to help dispel common nutrition myths and provide clarity on many nutrition-related topics.

Jenna Hope

HOW TO STAY HEALTHY

The nutritionist's guide
to optimising your immunity

PIATKUS

PIATKUS

First published in Great Britain in 2023 by Piatkus

5 7 9 10 8 6

Copyright © Jenna Hope 2023

The moral right of the author has been asserted.

A CIP catalogue record for this book
is available from the British Library.

ISBN: 978-0-349-43855-9

Typeset in Sabon by Hewer Text UK Ltd, Edinburgh
Printed and bound in Great Britain by Clays Ltd, Elcograf S.p.A.

Papers used by Piatkus are from well-managed forests and other responsible sources.

Piatkus
An imprint of
Little, Brown Book Group
Carmelite House
50 Victoria Embankment
London EC4Y 0DZ

An Hachette UK Company
www.hachette.co.uk

www.littlebrown.co.uk

Contents

Introduction

Have you ever really thought about your role in supporting the most fundamental system which supports you . . . the immune system? I don't mean the times you're feeling run-down, when you might pop a vitamin C supplement or snack on an extra orange; what I'm really asking is whether you have ever considered how your everyday dietary and lifestyle behaviours impact your immunity? The immune system is one that is often undervalued and disregarded until we experience our first sniff or cough of the season. At that point we're likely to stock up on lemons, honey, vitamin C supplements and boxes of tissues. However, the immune system is complex and plays a significantly greater role in our everyday health than just fighting off winter colds and flu. It is the body's defence mechanism and it's working 24/7, constantly warding off unwanted pathogens. As you turn the pages of this book, your immune system is working behind the scenes to help keep you safe and well.

What is now becoming clear is that the food that we're consuming, the lifestyles we're leading and the activities we're engaging in can all contribute to helping or hindering the immune system to perform its job optimally.

Over the past four years we've developed more awareness of the role of our immune systems, as they have come under serious threat from the Covid-19 pandemic in the world around us. The truth is, however, prior to 2020 – and even now as our memory of the pandemic dwindles – many of us didn't give a second thought to our immune system. It took me twenty-one years until I even considered the simple fact that my immune system could save my life (it is, in fact, saving our lives every minute of every day). While this may sound dramatic, four weeks in hospital with an MRSA infection really helped me to understand and be grateful for my immune system. I was in my third year at university studying nutrition, but until that point I hadn't truly appreciated the role of the immune system and how it protects us. Thankfully (as I'm still here, writing this book), my immune system kicked into gear, with the help of modern medicine, and I left the hospital with a deeper drive to further understand our health and motivate others to optimise their everyday wellbeing. That experience taught me that it's not what we do today or tomorrow for our wellbeing that's important, it's what we do time and time again, day in and day out. This way we can support our long-term health and wellbeing when it really matters the most.

Considering our immune health really is our key to life – and a healthy one at that. It's surprising that as a population we don't take more notice or care of it on a daily basis. In this book, I'm going to share a wide range of tips and tricks that will benefit your immunity and your health on a day-to-day basis. This isn't about 'boosting' your immune system: as we'll explore later, this term and approach can sometimes cause more harm than good. It's about providing the immune system with the necessary tools to be able to function optimally. However, my approach is slightly different. Rather than boosting the immune system when we feel it may need it, I believe we need to support it on a day-to-day basis. We're all busy enough and often have far more on our plates than we can handle, so I'm not here to provide you with more work, ask you to purchase expensive and unnecessary concoctions, or to overwhelm you with unachievable 'must-dos'. I'm here to demonstrate how small but effective changes can transform your life and optimise your immunity and improve your physical and overall wellbeing. Feel free to dip in and out of this book as a guide when you need it, or you can read it from cover to cover; however, reading the first five chapters consecutively will give you an understanding of how the immune system works and what its individual components are, which will relate to the more practical tips and tricks I share in later chapters.

Before we dive into the subject, I want to share a little bit about my approach to nutrition, which really sits at the heart of this book and the advice that I'll be sharing with you. I'm a Registered Nutritionist, wife, daughter, sister, mummy (currently in waiting but hopefully by the time of publication it will be official) and an avid foodie. I often encounter the perception that being a nutritionist means you don't really enjoy food and view it as solely serving a functional purpose. However, this is a complete misconception! When I was growing up, food was always a major part of my life, my daily routine and family get-togethers. My mother tells me that as a baby I was never interested in milk but from day one of weaning, as soon as the highchair came out, the bib went on and the food was put down, my arms would flap and the excitement was real. I'm proud to say that although I've lost the highchair, the bib and the flapping arms along the way, my excitement and enthusiasm towards every meal since has remained the same.

While I'm no cordon bleu chef, I am a cooking enthusiast and I get great pleasure from experimenting with new foods, flavours and dishes, and sharing my love of food with others. The best

part of all of this joy is the knowledge that you can simultaneously get so much pleasure from the simple act of eating while
nourishing your body and your immune system.

So, rest assured, this book isn't going to encourage you to drop
your favourite foods or even tell you to add a portion of broccoli to
every meal; it's about inspiring you to nourish your immune system
through a wide range of dietary and lifestyle habits. We both know
that not every piece of advice in this book is going to tick all your
boxes and that's OK. It's about discovering those habits that will
work for you and those that you feel are the most achievable.

The number one rule in my clinic, and that is the basis for
every piece of work I've ever done, is that food should be delicious
and nutritious and – most importantly – incredibly satisfying.
In the pages that follow, I'll walk you through a breakdown of
the science of the immune system and the science of nutrition;
I'll share my most practical tips for how you can incorporate
the science into your everyday life; and I'll share a variety of
immune-friendly recipes to help encourage and empower you to
make positive changes to your diet, which will reignite your love
of food while supporting your immunity. The recipes in Chapter
11 are based on a variety of delicious flavours and ingredients,
alluring colours and diverse textures and I really hope you find
the pleasure in them too.

So that's enough about who I am and my passion for food and
nutrition, let's drill down to some more serious issues.

In the UK we're blessed with a healthcare service that is free
at the point of use and one which we're incredibly fortunate to
be able to access. The doctors, nurses, midwives, healthcare
assistants, dietitians and everyone who works for the NHS do
an incredible job.

Yet it's no secret that our NHS is in crisis and, due to the nature of funding, it operates on a 'cure over prevention' basis. Consequently, as a nation, we're more likely to focus on managing ill health than preventing it in the first place. There's no doubt that there are many illnesses which we may not be able to prevent through diet and lifestyle alone but there are so many more that we can. The aim of this book is not to negate the power of modern medicine – which we are extremely lucky to have access to – but to show that it needn't always necessarily be the first port of call. In Chapter 10, I'll share some top tips about how you can manage your immune system when you feel it's under attack. You'll see that it's not always about reaching straight for medication. Furthermore, understanding the role that our diet and lifestyle plays in supporting our immune system is the perfect place to start to work towards a prevention over cure approach. If we can make just a few small positive changes, whether to our daily activities and routines or to the foods that are regularly passing our lips, we're sure to set ourselves on the right path towards prevention rather than cure. It's not about getting it right 100 per cent of the time, it's about doing our best with the resources that we have. I really hope that this book will become an invaluable resource that will help you nourish your immunity in a bid for a healthy body and lifestyle.

In the first two chapters I'll introduce the importance of health and nutrition, and the immune system and its individual components, to highlight how it really works, before going on to explore the role of the gut on our immune health. The gut is an organ that in recent years has gained a lot of attention online and in the media. However, there are many misinterpretations of its role, how it works and what we can do to nurture it daily, so I'll be sharing the truths and the tips on how to optimise the function of your gut too. In Chapter 4, I explain the role of our early lives on our immunity (although feel free to skip this part if this doesn't feel as relevant to you).

We'll then deep dive into the nutrients required to support your immune health before looking at the key dietary and life-style behaviours that impact our immunity. I'll walk you through the foods that we want to increase in our diets and those we should be aiming to reduce. Additionally, we'll explore the influence of a wide range of activities on the immune system. I'll be answering all of those burning questions too: how much coffee can I drink? Should I be taking probiotics? What supplements should I be taking? Is cold-water therapy really helpful? And so many more. I'll also explore dietary approaches in relation to autoimmune conditions and in Chapter 11 you'll find some pull-out pages to support you through the times when your immune system has come under fire.

What You Can Expect From This Book

I've written this book in the hope that it will inspire and empower you to make healthier dietary and lifestyle decisions to support your immunity. Despite that, this isn't about overhauling your whole life or letting your diet take complete control of your thoughts and behaviours. It's about making small but consistent changes every day to set yourself up for the future. Your immune system is an important key which can help unlock a healthier future and if we do our best to nourish it every day then we'll be doing a great job. I'll discuss a whole host of topics and factors which influence our immune system and it's for you to decide which ones you're most interested in, what you want to take on board and what you want to leave on the page. Remember, we're all individual and what works for one person may not be practical or beneficial for another. Additionally, while the information is directed towards supporting a healthier immune system you're likely to see benefits which go far beyond your immunity. You can expect some well-explained science (fear not, it's more than manageable), the theories behind healthier living and some practical tips and tricks to encourage you to begin to implement these changes today. Nothing I tell you will be too obscure, too expensive or highly impractical. I'm all about smart, simple and sustainable nutrition. I commit to equipping you with the most effective and pragmatic tips and tools; all I ask from you is that you make the commitment to improve your wellbeing in any way you can (no matter how big or how small). I promise you it will be worth it.

Now is the time for you to think about what you want to achieve from reading this book and why you picked it up in the first place. If you can keep that motivation with you as you read through the pages you're far more likely to get the most from this book.

So, grab a cup of herbal tea, get comfortable and feel free to scribble over the pages as you decide which tips you'd love to adopt to support your immune health and your general wellbeing on a daily basis. Are you ready to feel the best version of yourself (and I really mean that)?

CHAPTER 1

Introduction to Nutrition and Health

What Is Health?

What does health mean to you? Take a pause for a moment and really think about the answer to this. You may even want to write it down and come back to it as you read the rest of this book.

Whatever the official definitions of health might be, we're all going to have a completely different take on what health means to us and why our health is important. This awareness can often be used as the driving factor to encourage behaviour change.

In 1984 the World Health Organization defined health as: 'a state of complete physical, mental and social wellbeing and not merely the absence of disease or infirmity'. This has since become somewhat controversial as the definition suggests that we can't live a healthy life alongside a chronic disease, yet clearly there are many individuals who do live with chronic diseases and who may argue otherwise. However, specifics of the definition aside, it's the words *physical, mental and social* which are the most important. In the past we've commonly thought of health in relation to our physical wellbeing. It's not been until recent decades that the topic of mental health has gathered pace to appear at the top of social consciousness. As a result, this conversation is being opened up more routinely and we're far more aware of the impact of mental health on physical wellbeing. In spite of this, our social wellbeing is an area of health that often still gets left behind; however, when thinking about our dietary and lifestyle approaches in supporting physical and mental health, it's absolutely crucial that we don't forget about the social implications of our decisions and our behaviours. Let's dig a little deeper into what this looks like in reality, using diet as an example.

Throughout my career I've constantly been asked the question, 'What is the perfect diet?' My answer will always remain the same: the truth is the perfect diet does not exist. A perfect diet on paper may well be one that optimises your physical wellbeing or supports your immune system. However, going back to the three categories of wellbeing associated with good health – physical, mental and social – the sacrifices that come with consuming a diet designed for physical perfection often mean that you're missing out on all the other benefits associated with food. For example, you might regularly be skipping a catch-up with friends over a glass of wine or always saying no to a natter over a coffee and a slice of cake. By depriving yourself of the many things that can bring you joy, you might find that you're neglecting your mental and social health at the expense of following a 'perfect' diet.

Why does this matter? It matters because evidence consistently shows that deprivation can contribute to an increase in the desire for these foods or drinks and, as a result, you're more likely to end up consuming them in excess. These feelings of deprivation – and often isolation – can leave you feeling miserable, guilty and unmotivated, which can therefore contribute to a more negative mental state. In such cases, your dietary and lifestyle decisions may start to dictate your social behaviours and you may find yourself turning down parties or social events if there's nothing you can eat, or the timings don't suit your dietary plan. On these occasions our social wellbeing is far more important than we often give credit to. Loneliness is increasingly becoming an area of interest since evidence has highlighted that as the incidence of loneliness increases so does an individual's perception of any present chronic illnesses. It's for this reason that our social wellbeing is pivotal to our immune health, general physical health and mental wellbeing.

This example is just one of many that shows how important it is to consider the social, mental and physical aspects of our health when thinking about how we can adopt a healthier lifestyle. But there are many other factors which can influence our overall wellbeing too. These include sleep health, sexual health, financial health, environmental health, family set-ups, relationships and lifestyles – all major players in the picture of complete health.

Now that we've looked at the importance of considering our health in a more holistic way, let's return to the question I asked at the start of this chapter: what does health mean to you? Has your answer changed? It's OK if it hasn't, but if it has carry this thought with you as you read through the pages to come.

Alongside having a deep-rooted gratitude for my immune system, my interpretation of health is one in which I can efficiently carry out my everyday tasks feeling as energised, positive and motivated as possible. I've by no means got everything nailed down to a tee, yet my own version of health encourages me to consume nourishing foods on a daily basis while still allowing me to relish a glass (or two) of rosé at a summer barbecue or a mug of mulled wine by the fire in the winter. I thoroughly enjoy long walks in nature with my nearest and dearest and Dora, our border collie, but also love curling up on the sofa after a long day in clinic. I really appreciate the role my friends and family play in my social wellbeing and can always rely on them to recharge my social battery where necessary. All of our interpretations look different and mine is just one example of the many ways to view health. Whatever your personal interpretation is, I think we can all agree that our health is our most critical resource, one which we require throughout our everyday lives. No matter how successful we are in life, if we don't have our health then it's arguable that we're not really living life to its optimum potential.

Once we've identified what health means to us and why it's important, the next question is: who is really responsible for our health? It's common to believe that there are many factors that play a role in the responsibility for our health. Our governments are often an easy target, along with the food industry (arguably an even easier one). But there is also the NHS, the education system, genetics, upbringing and childhood experiences, societal norms, those we surround ourselves with and some might say even our employers can play a role. There's no question that all of these components are involved but, ultimately, taking responsibility for looking after our *own* health can be so much more empowering and achievable. Once we acknowledge that we do have the power, we're often far more able to make the changes that we so desire. (Although I'm definitely not suggesting it's an easy task.)

To caveat this, there are of course cases where the determining factors of our health lie beyond our control (for example, in the hands a medical professional, as a result of an accident or because of a genetic or medical predisposition). By suggesting that we take responsibility for our health I'm by no means underestimating the challenges which we can face in doing so. I am, however, suggesting that shifting the responsibility to those who hold some level of influence is often unhelpful and unconstructive. As we take responsibility and we make changes, we'll all face our own individual and unique challenges but I hope that some of the information and practical tips in this book will play a role in helping to equip you with the knowledge and desire to look after your wellbeing and immunity in a way that is achievable.

What Does a Healthy Lifestyle Look Like?

A healthy lifestyle is often dressed up as a picture that encompasses drinking daily green juices, engaging in yoga multiple times per week, hitting the gym hard and coming home to a fresh bowl of salad. This may well be a healthy lifestyle for some people but for the majority of us it's about feeling energised, socially fulfilled, with good sleep patterns and positive mental health. To me a salubrious lifestyle is all about balance, self-fulfilment and setting myself up for a healthy future. You, however, may have a totally different view of what a healthy lifestyle looks like for you and because we are all unique that's to be expected. The key is that you feel well, energised and happy, and that your lifestyle is working for you rather than against you.

What Is Nutrition?

While health and nutrition are often used in synergy, the definition of nutrition is significantly different to the one of health. Nutrition is defined as 'the process of providing or obtaining the food necessary for health and growth'. It's a multi-faceted approach to how elements in food can provide the necessary nourishment for the maintenance of life. I think it's important to take a holistic approach to nutrition as we need to consider the impacts of our dietary choices from a molecular level right up to a societal level – as well as everything in between. Nutrition can be used to optimise health and wellbeing while also contributing to reducing the risks of illness and disease.

Alongside many other health and lifestyle behaviours, nutrition plays a powerful role in supporting our everyday health, wellbeing and our immune function, but it's important to note that nutrition alone is certainly not the panacea to health. Nutrition science is an area of constant scientific evolvement as we're continually widening our understanding of nutrients, nutrient interactions, dietary patterns, the influences which are driving our dietary choices and how all of this impacts our physical and mental wellbeing. It's also easy to be thrown off course by the common misconceptions and misinformation about nutrition that have surfaced as interest in the topic has widened over the last few decades. Anecdotal evidence often drives many nutrition myths and it's important to remember that the experiences of just one or two people is not enough to promote long-term, responsible nutrition recommendations. Human nutrition is a very complex science and often the answers may not always be as straightforward as we'd like. In the chapters to follow I'll do my best to make it as easily actionable and digestible as possible to allow you to use nutrition in order to support your health and optimise your immunity.

What Is the Role of Nutrition in Our Health?

I grew up in the nineties and if you recall this time, you'll likely remember that size zero celebrities were regularly plastered over the front pages of every magazine and when their size changed we were sure to be told about it. It's no wonder we were left thinking about food in relation to just one thing . . . weight. I have to credit my mum here who actually brought us up with the idea that healthy food was about maintaining heart health. I've since learned that there's much more to nutrition and food than just the cardiovascular aspect, but nonetheless it was an excellent distraction from the weight-focused society in which I and many others grew up. Since the nineties it's promising to see that we've stepped away from the sole focus that nutrition is simply about a number on the scale and that it's now understood that it plays far more of a critical role on our overall wellbeing. Nutrition has a vital impact on our health, development and growth and these effects occur long before we even enter the world: evidence now shows that the maternal diet prior to conception and throughout pregnancy can set up a child's nutrition status for later on in life. (We'll discuss this in more detail in Chapter 4.)

Some of the ways in which nutrition has the power to impact our physical health include supporting normal growth, the immune system and good sleep and slowing down the ageing process, plus it can help to reduce the risks of developing many non-communicable diseases (those which can't be transferred between individuals). Some examples of non-communicable diseases include type 2 diabetes, cardiovascular disease, arthritis and types of lung diseases to name just a few. Yet, it also has the power to impact our psychological health, helping us to manage stress, low mood and a lack of motivation. The social impact of nutrition stretches far beyond a glass of wine or slice of cake with a friend. It has long been an integral component of our society, from religious gatherings and family occasions to sports competitions and social engagements. Food is often used as a way to express our love, gratitude and appreciation for others. In my house, growing up, food was a central component of the way in which my family came together: on both joyous and sombre occasions our love and support was expressed through food. It's for this reason that I am so passionate that while food should (for the most part) be nourishing and healthy it should first and foremost always be enjoyable and satisfying.

So although I'm not suggesting that the effect of food on body weight isn't important (it absolutely has a place), it's far from the total picture. Throughout the rest of the book you'll see just how influential nutrition can be on other areas of our general health, but particularly in supporting our immunity.

Why Should We Care About Our Nutrition and Health?

I suspect the very fact that you picked up this book suggests that you already have the answer to this question. Evidently our health sits at the epicentre of our wellbeing. Without it we struggle to support an optimal quality of life and if we're not focusing on good health, eventually we're sure to experience ill health. If we're supporting our immune system and our health on a daily basis, it's much more likely to support us when we need it most. If we're constantly engaging in behaviours that neglect the immune system (and our health) then we can't expect that same immune system to be working optimally when required.

The strongest form of motivation is intrinsic; this is when you have a true internal desire to make changes in order to optimise long-term health. However, for some people the motivation to change their diet or lifestyle and to focus on their health can frequently come from an extrinsic source, where you are focused on a particular external outcome or an external reward. The key part is that you have a genuine requirement and drive to improve your quality of life or maintain your levels of good health. I hope that as you read through this book, your desire to make healthier changes to your diet and lifestyle develops. I can assure you that once you notice the impact of making healthier choices the drive to continue making positive decisions will continue to strengthen.

Summary Points

- Health is defined as 'a state of complete physical, mental and social wellbeing and not merely the absence of disease or infirmity', although our own definition will be unique to each of us.
- Nutrition plays a vital role in the development and future of our health, growth and immune system.
- The food we eat has the power to impact our physical health in a number of ways.

- The roles of food extend far beyond nourishing our body and can play an important part in supporting our mental and social wellbeing too. Food helps to bring people together and is often used as a way to express emotion between individuals.
- A healthy lifestyle is one which leaves you feeling physically energised, positive and thriving most of the time, although it's important to nourish our social and mental wellbeing too.

CHAPTER 2

Introduction to Immunity

Now that we've looked at the role of nutrition in our overall health, we're moving on to explore the fundamentals of the immune system to allow us to marry nutrition and immunity later on in the book. As we've explored, the food we eat directly impacts all areas of our health and the immune system is no different; it's fuelled by the nutrients which we consume daily. In this chapter we'll dive into the intricacies of the immune system and how it works. We'll explore the different layers within our immune system and the roles of the specific cells in this system. This chapter will help to set the scene and provide a background for the more practical advice in the later chapters. I think it's important to fully understand why we're being given certain advice as the why is often a factor which encourages us to buy into making healthier dietary and lifestyle changes. As we explored in the introduction, considering the significant role the immune system has to play on our everyday functioning it's barely given enough time in the spotlight. This is its time to shine and for you to fully explore and appreciate how the immune system works to enable you to support and optimise it every day.

What Is the Immune System?

The immune system is a hugely complex system of processes and organs in the body, which help to protect us against infections and diseases.

Much like in an army where all the soldiers have different roles, there are many different components within the immune system, each playing a distinct role.

The barriers

The first component of the immune system comprises the barriers between our internal and external environment. These include the nose, the skin, the eyes, the mouth, the genito-urinary tract and the digestive tract (the 9-metre long tube which runs from the mouth to the colon). As all of these areas have entry points to the body, it's important that they have their own mechanisms for defence.

Our eyes are a strong barrier for defence as they contain our tear fluid. This has antibacterial properties and is constantly flushing the eyeballs of unwanted intruders every time we blink. In the mouth we have tonsils (unless they've been removed) and saliva. The tonsils act as a barrier to prevent foreign pathogens entering the digestive tract and the salvia contains antibacterial properties to help fight intruders too. The tonsils are often one of the first points of contact for an intruder; they're constantly working hard to fight against pathogens and consequently are vulnerable to becoming overwhelmed. As a result, infection of the tonsils, also known as tonsillitis, is prevalent. (If you were particularly prone to tonsillitis you may well have had your tonsils removed, but this isn't a cause for concern as we have many other defence mechanisms to protect us.) In the nose we have nasal hairs and mucus, which can prevent unwanted pathogens from passing through the nasal passage, into the body and along the digestive tract. We have hydrochloric acid in the stomach which can contribute to destroying nasty organisms that have been ingested. Furthermore, the gut lining and the gut microbes also play a fundamental role in protecting the body from unwanted pathogens (I'll discuss the gut in more detail in Chapter 3).

The immune cells

The immune system is also made up of immune cells, the most common being white blood cells. These white blood cells, also known as leukocytes, are located all around the body in the blood, bone marrow, skeletal muscle, skin cells and our organs. If any unwanted pathogens pass through the barriers discussed above, then the white blood cells act as the next line of defence.

On average, a healthy individual will create between 80 and 100 billion new white blood cells every single day. Collectively they play a vital role in identifying and destroying unwanted pathogens and mediating the inflammatory response. There are a variety of main types of white blood cells, all of which have unique characteristics.

Types of white blood cells (leukocytes)

- **Neutrophils (the First Responders)** These cells are the first on the scene and make up more of the white blood cells than any of the other types of leukocytes. They're able to reach the targeted site fast and can help in

blocking invading pathogens from moving further into
the body.

- **Monocytes (the Cleaning Agents)** These cells help to
  break down the unwanted bacteria and clean up any cells
  that may have been destroyed.
- **Lymphocytes (the Fighters)** These cells fight and attack
  the unwanted bacteria and pathogens. These include
  T-lymphocytes, B-lymphocytes and natural killer cells,
  all of which we will explore later in more detail.
- **Basophils (the Alarm Bells)** The role of these cells is to
  generate the alert that there's an intruder; they produce
  histamine, which creates the allergic responses such
  as coughing and sneezing that we're all familiar with.
  Coughing and sneezing have a vital role in attempting
  to eliminate the unwanted pathogens.
- **Eosinophils (the Reserve Fighters)** These cells help to
  attack and kill parasites that the other cells may not be
  able to handle alone.

There are many factors which can impact the number of white
blood cells we have circulating at any given time. Common
causes of a low white blood cell count (a risk factor for infection) can include bone marrow failure, leukaemia, some drugs
such as chemotherapy and vitamin B12 deficiency – to name
just a few. On the other hand, common causes of a high white
blood cell count can include viral or bacterial infections as well
as autoimmune conditions. This is often seen in those who are
particularly prone to infections. Measuring your white blood
cell count can often be done via a full blood count test by your
doctor, so if you are concerned about your white blood cell
count or any aspect of your health and wellbeing it's always

advised that you seek help from your general practitioner or healthcare professional.

The lymphatic system

The next component is the lymphatic system. Our lymphatic organs (the lymph nodes, bone marrow and spleen) are an integral part of the immune system. The lymph nodes help to capture the unwanted bacteria and viruses alongside helping to store some of the immune cells. We have hundreds of lymph nodes located all over the body and they're often found in locations to help them identify invaders. Lymph nodes are commonly referred to as glands and it's not uncommon for them to swell up when the immune system is under attack: we're all likely to have experienced our 'glands being up' at some point in our lives. The bone marrow and the spleen are the organs which regularly produce and differentiate new immune cells that can be deployed around the body. These are produced via stem cells, which are readily found in the bone marrow.

Cytokines

Additionally, we have molecules known as cytokines, which are another significant component of our immune system. Cytokines are produced by the T-cells (a type of lymphocyte) and are chemical messengers which help to regulate the immune and inflammatory responses. They're also often used as a biomarker of inflammation in the body and are measured through the blood. Cytokines can be proinflammatory or anti-inflammatory depending on the context, the situation and the need and therefore they work on both sides of supporting immune function.

The Immune Response

There are two key stages in the immune response: stage one involves what's known as the innate immune system, and stage two involves the adaptive immune system.

The primary role of the innate immune system is to respond quickly, and as such it uses the same tools and mechanisms to respond to every foreign substance or perceived attacker which it's exposed to. This means that while it is quick and efficient, it doesn't have the ability or the time to identify pathogens and respond in the most effective or accurate way. As a result, the potential of the innate immune system is quite limited. Once an intruder has made its way past the skin, or any of the entry points and mucous membranes, and into the body, the innate immune system triggers an initial, local inflammatory response. Common symptoms of this response can include swelling, redness, discomfort, pain and rashes. Once this initial response has been triggered, you may also experience other typical symptoms such as a temperature, headache, fever or fatigue that last a few days while your body works to fight and protect against the intruder. We often perceive these symptoms to be a negative but it's important to remember that these are often a sign that our immune system is working effectively.

However, when the innate immune system is unable to deal with the intruder on its own, the adaptive immune system will take over to carry out the next steps in the defence sequence. The adaptive immune system does exactly as it says on the tin: it adapts over time and in response to our exposures and experiences. Before launching in, the adaptive immune system spends a bit more time observing and attempting to identify the pathogen to see if it recognises it. While this means the adaptive immune system may take longer to kick into gear, it allows it to be able to build up a bank of knowledge of different pathogens to better deal with them over time and – more specifically – if they were to intrude again, the adaptive immune system can work faster. The adaptive immune system is predominantly run by the lymphocytes (which we met earlier), specifically two types: T-lymphocytes (T-cells) and B-lymphocytes (B-cells). The T-cells are produced in the bone marrow and are then carried via the blood to the thymus gland, where they are able to develop and mature to ensure they're ready for action. These T-cells have three main roles: they are responsible for detecting cells that have been damaged by the intruder, identifying the unwanted pathogens and then sending chemical messages to the T-helper cells who can then assist on the scene too. In addition, they also work with the B-cells to generate a memory of the unwanted pathogen. This ensures that if the same pathogen returns again, the T-cells can quickly multiply to produce a strong response to help protect us against an illness or infection.

Ideally, over time, your body develops a quicker and stronger response to the pathogens which it already recognises. However, a weakened or compromised immune system can impact our ability to recognise and fight off the same intruder time and time again.

I've explained the two phases of the immune response; however, when the immune system is under fire the innate and adaptive immune cells often work in conjunction with each other in order to target the intruders. It's the collaborative approach which produces the most successful outcomes. As with everything in the world of health and nutrition, it's important to remember that we are all completely different; while there are multiple factors that impact our uniqueness and more spe-cifically the individuality of our immune systems, it's the slight differences in our T-cells and B-cells that play a significant role in affecting how strong we are at fighting off unwanted pathogens.

The uniqueness of our immune systems is a critical factor in our evolution and resilience as a species. If we were all identical, with exactly the same immune system, there would be a far greater likelihood that an individual pathogen would be able to infect us all, which consequently could wipe out a large number of our species relatively quickly.

Earlier, I touched on inflammation, which is a reaction caused by a response from the immune system. Although often uncomfortable, this is a necessary part of the immune response as it helps to highlight the site of the infection and is a key indicator that the immune cells are functioning properly. It is often given a bad rap and carries a lot of negative connotations. Nowadays supermarket shelves are brimming with products making extreme anti-inflammatory promises and claiming to be the magic cure for inflammation.

As with many things in life, inflammation has its pros and cons. It is actually a very critical component of the immune system. The inflammatory response described above is what's known as an acute response, meaning it's stimulated for a short period of time and for a specific task. A well-functioning immune system is incredibly smart and once the role of inflammation has been fulfilled, the system releases another type of T-cells, known as T-regulatory cells, and also anti-inflammatory cytokines, both of which are responsible for activating the anti-inflammatory response. To give you an example, when you get stung by a bee or a wasp the site of the sting can become sore, red and inflamed, but once the immune cells have dealt with the unwanted pathogens the inflammation often decreases. However, the key is that we need to keep inflammation as contained and as acute as possible.

Keeping T-regulatory cells in a fine equilibrium is really important for ensuring the immune system can work optimally. If we have too few T-regulatory cells we wouldn't be able to downregulate the immune system, which can mean that if left to its own devices the immune cells could start to attack our friendly cells; this can creep into autoimmune territory (which I'll discuss in more detail later). However, if we have too many T-regulatory cells, the immune system response may be suppressed before the job is complete, meaning the intruders could be left with unrestricted access.

This level of acute inflammation may not necessarily impact our everyday quality of life. However, sometimes chronic low-level inflammation can lead to a very slow journey to ill health. Chronic inflammation is a significant driving factor in a variety of non-communicable diseases. Later on, I'll come back to how you can support your health and immune system for the long term and how to help reduce chronic inflammation through your diet and lifestyle practices.

Why Our Immune Systems Are All Different

Some scientists have suggested that our immune systems are as unique as our fingerprints and, as I suggested earlier, this may be to ensure that we're able to withstand a variety of viruses and bacteria thereby increasing the resilience and longevity of the human race.

The male vs female immune systems

Over the years that my husband and I have been together (eight years and counting), I've become very familiar with the term 'man-flu'. This is a term which is used in our house each time my husband catches a sniffle. I can't be the only one who struggles to pander to the idea of 'man-flu'. However, as much as I hate to admit it, the research does show that immune systems really do differ between the sexes.

While there may be a few reasons for these variations, it does appear that the difference in our hormones and our chromosomes may be two very significant factors. Oestrogen and progesterone have been found to be the key hormones that contribute to the differences between the male and female immune systems. Oestrogen is a hormone which is generally present in much higher levels in females than in males (although males do have some too). It has been shown to increase the strength of the immune cells and their ability to release cytokines (the chemical messengers which play a role in regulating the inflammatory and the immune responses). The immune system has a number of hormone receptors throughout the body, meaning that the immune cells are able to respond to the higher levels of oestrogen and progesterone. This may be a reason why these hormones can help to strengthen the responses of the immune system. In support of the hormone theory, studies have also shown the presence of testosterone and androgens (both of which are generally higher in post-pubescent men) have been associated with a suppression in immune cell activity and a reduction in natural killer cells (a type of white blood cell).

Another contributing factor to the differences in the immune systems are our chromosomes. It's believed that the X chromosomes have a significantly higher number of genes related to the regulation of the immune response when compared with the Y chromosomes. Since males have XY chromosomes and females have XX chromosomes, females therefore may have a much greater number of immune-related genes. This may also be a contributing factor as to why generally females have a higher life expectancy than males. Furthermore, females are likely to respond better to vaccinations than males. For those female readers who may be thinking that this sounds really promising and that we're the stronger sex when it comes to immunity, it's not necessarily all positive news. While it's true that a stronger immune system in females can mean that we're able to fight viruses and unwanted bacteria faster than a male's immune system, an immune system which is *too* strong can pose an increased risk of autoimmune disorders. In fact, research suggests that 80 per cent of individuals with autoimmune disorders are female.

In later chapters, I'll dive deeper into other factors which can positively and negatively impact our immune system. However, the research does suggest that environmental and dietary factors can affect the male and female immune systems differently. There are also suggestions that these differences between males and females can change depending on our age and our reproductive status. It's also important to highlight that your sex alone does not predetermine the fate of your immune system; there are many more pieces to the jigsaw.

The Role of the Immune System in Allergies

You may not necessarily automatically associate the immune system with an allergy but the two are very much interlinked, as the symptoms of an allergy are the immune system's response to a specific substance. When we're exposed to an allergen, the immune system responds by attacking the substance and treating it as an intruder. Often the response is immediate; symptoms can include swelling of tissues, a runny nose, wheezing and appearance of a rash or itching. The immune response to an allergen can vary greatly with some being rather mild and manageable and others posing a risk of a life-threating anaphylactic shock. Symptoms of anaphylaxis include drastic swelling of tissues, difficulty breathing, tightness in the throat or chest, nausea and headaches and severe itching.

A person can be allergic to almost any substance, although common allergens include various foods, pollen, grass, dust mites and some medications. Often common allergies such as these initiate an IgE mediated response, which is where the immune system produces specific immunoglobulin E antibodies. In such cases, the allergic response is rather instant and can present in the form of sneezing, an immediate presentation of a rash or – in severe cases – difficulty breathing. These responses can be stimulated by a very small exposure to the substance. However, some allergies can be non-IgE mediated; in such cases, it can take up to 24 hours for the allergic symptoms to present themselves and may require exposures to higher doses to be triggered. These allergies still initiate a response from the immune cells but they do not involve the production of immunoglobulin E antibodies and can be therefore more challenging to identify and understand. The symptoms of these can include changes to bowel movements (diarrhoea, vomiting and abdominal discomfort) or rashes and changes to the skin.

There's a common misconception that we're born with allergies, but we can in fact develop them (and grow out of them) at any stage of life. Some individuals may be more predisposed to allergies due to a family history or specific genes that can increase the risk of developing an allergy.

The prevalence of allergies in the UK is believed to be increasing and it's thought that our diets and lifestyles can contribute to these increases. For example, high levels of stress, our obsessions with cleaning products and antibacterial products and high intakes of sugars and saturated fats are just a few of the factors contributing to increasing the risks of allergies.

IgE-mediated allergies are often diagnosed through skin prick tests and, generally speaking, avoiding the allergen is often the only way to manage the allergy. That said, modern developments have shown that allergy immunotherapy or allergy desensitisation can be highly effective in treating allergies in some individuals. These techniques should only ever be conducted under the guidance of a medical professional.

The terms allergy and intolerance are often used interchangeably, although they do not produce the same immune response. Unlike food allergies, food intolerances do not involve the immune system and are less harmful and dangerous than allergies, although they can have a disadvantageous effect on an individual's lifestyle, physical comfort and mental wellbeing. For example, if you're constantly worried about the discomfort caused from consuming a certain food this may stop you enjoying meals out, contributing to stress and anxiety around eating. Unlike a food allergy, the 'tolerance level' in those with a food intolerance can be much higher. For example, if someone is allergic to gluten, even the slightest contamination (for example, using a knife that has just been used to cut gluten-containing bread) could bring on an immune response. However, an individual with an intolerance to gluten is likely to be able to tolerate such a small amount of exposure to the substance without experiencing symptoms.

It's important to differentiate between the two terms as overusing the term allergy when referring to an intolerance can devalue the importance of avoiding cross-contamination and exposures to potential allergens. If you are concerned about a food allergy or an intolerance it's best to seek advice from your GP or healthcare professional.

The Hygiene Hypothesis vs the Old Friends Hypothesis

The Hygiene Hypothesis is a term coined by Dr David Stratchan in 1989. Through his observations Dr Stratchan identified a correlation between a reduced exposure to viruses and infection from older siblings throughout childhood and a higher incidence and risk of allergic disease in childhood and later on in life.

However, more recently, scientists have questioned the responsibility of the term 'hygiene hypothesis' as they fear that it could encourage people to neglect their personal hygiene and consequently encounter more of the negative effects of poor food hygiene, a lack of handwashing and reduced hygiene in the home. Since the traction of Dr Stratchan's original hypothesis, researchers are now suggesting that it may not be a case of being 'too clean' that is causing the rise in atopic diseases and autoimmune conditions, but it may in fact be a lack of early contact with the right type of microbial exposures. Atopic diseases are those which have a strong immune-related allergic response. They often have a genetic predisposition and include disorders such as asthma, allergic rhinitis and atopic eczema.

As a result of these concerns, the hygiene hypothesis has been re-termed as 'The Old Friends Hypothesis'. The 'right' types of exposures refer not to the viruses and diseases which were previously believed to have an immune-building purpose, but rather exposure to friendly bacteria in our environments. There are many theories as to why we may be less exposed to these 'right' microbes in the early years; these include our use of sanitised food and water, the overuse of antibiotics, general sanitation, an increase in personal hygiene and changes to our lifestyle which has seen a shift from a rural, farming lifestyle to one which is more urban. It's worth noting that many of these changes occurred over a relatively short period of time and therefore our immune systems haven't had sufficient time to evolve and make the necessary adaptations to deal with these changes. Consequently, it's the immune system which has since come under fire and for some people this is more problematic than for others.

While it's not necessarily clear exactly why our exposures to these microbes have diminished, there are a few factors which can impact the ability of the microbes to interact with and help to regulate the immune system. These include the type of microorganism exposure which we are deprived of, at what stage of our development we were deprived (e.g. pre-natal, neo-natal, early childhood or later in life), our individual genetic predisposition to atopic diseases and our individual dietary and lifestyle factors.

In more recent years, and since Covid-19, our hygiene has once again been overhauled and I can't help but question the long-term impact of social distancing, lockdowns, the overuse of antibacterial hand gel, sprays and the obsession with hygiene on our future immune health. This is by no means a criticism of our approach to hygiene or the protocols introduced during the Covid-19 pandemic. It was evidently necessary at the time; however, we have to question the long-term impact on our gut and our immune system of overusing antibacterial handwash and cleaning products. Are these products going to completely reduce our exposure to pathogens? While this may sound like they'd be having the desired effect, there's potentially an argument that in the long term a lack of exposure will inhibit our immune cells from adapting and responding accordingly.

A 2022 review also highlighted the concern around the increased risk of flu, colds and other viral infections as a result of our hygiene measures. However, it's suggested that it's not the lack of exposure to the Covid-19 SARS virus that has contributed to weakening the immune system, nor may it be that we're more susceptible to cold and flu post-pandemic due to a weakened immune system, but rather we may be more likely to experience the effects of these pathogens as we've had a significantly reduced exposure to these varieties of microbes for a prolonged period of time. In addition to this, the gut and the changes in our gut microbes due to the lack of social interaction could also be playing a role in our susceptibility to colds and flu. However, it is far too soon to be able to definitively say what impact the Covid-19 pandemic measures will have on our long-term immunity so for now these are simply theories that require further research.

Additionally, it's important to remember that the lack of exposure to specific microorganisms is only one piece of this pie. Since the original hygiene hypothesis, there have been many other theories as to why there may be an increase in the prevalence and the risk of allergic diseases. These go far beyond the idea that it's simply due to a lack of exposure to certain microbes. If we think about it, there are so many other changes which have occurred in our modern-day lifestyles that may also be contributing to the increased risk of allergic diseases. Many of these we will discuss in more detail later on, but to give you a very obvious example, our diets have changed drastically since the 1900s. The prevalence of dietary-related diseases such as obesity, metabolic syndrome and type 2 diabetes have shot up astronomically over the past decade and – unfortunately – aren't set to slow down. A recent report suggested that 50 per cent of the UK population will be overweight or obese by 2030. This has ramifications for our immune systems because obesity has long been associated with an increased risk of low-grade systemic inflammation. Therefore this projection is concerning, not only for the health of the individual but because of the increased stress and pressure which will be placed on the NHS as a result.

Furthermore, dietary changes have led to an increase in the risk of nutrient deficiencies, which may also be contributing to the rise in atopic diseases. You may be thinking *How can nutritional deficiencies be an issue in a population where the levels of overweight and obesity are higher than ever before?* The answer is simple: it's absolutely possible and unfortunately not uncommon to see malnutrition in overweight and obesity. The western diet is typically high in ultra-processed foods, sugar, salt and saturated fats. These foods are generally lower in micronutrients due to the artificial ingredients and ultra-processing methods which are required to make them. In addition to our dietary changes, our lifestyles are more stressful than ever before and stress (discussed in detail in Chapter 9) can also play a major role in disrupting everything from our gut microbiome, hormone function, sleep and dietary intakes to our immune cell function.

Can We Boost Our Immune System?

You only have to walk down the supermarket aisles to find products promising to boost your immune system, but is this really possible? A healthy immune system is working around the clock fighting off unwanted pathogens, yet it's often not until we start to feel under the weather that we're even aware of it. It's a highly complex system that requires a delicate balance of all its individual components in order for it to work effectively. It's incredibly difficult to over-activate one aspect of the immune system through diet alone. However, with the use of high-dose supplements it's feasible to knock the immune system out of balance and an overactivated immune system can actually *increase* the risk of autoimmune conditions. Therefore, boosting the immune system is not something to strive for; instead, I prefer to focus on the idea of supporting it and providing it with all the necessary components for it to work in unison and in equilibrium.

In the next chapter we're going to look at the relationship between the gut and the immune system, how the two interact and why it is such a central component in supporting healthy immune cells. We'll explore the individual components of the gut and how we can use diet and lifestyle to support them.

Summary Points

- The skin, eyes, nose and mouth are important components in the first line of defence. They each contain unique barriers to help ward off unwanted pathogens.
- The immune system comprises two layers, the innate immune system and the adaptive immune system.
- The innate immune system is the 'first responder' on the scene and behaves quickly and efficiently, although the response is not targeted to individual pathogens.
- The adaptive immune system is predominantly run by the T-cells and the B-cells. The adaptive immune system provides a more specialised and targeted response to individual intruders.
- The adaptive immune system can remember unwanted pathogens and create antibodies, which can help to protect against repeated intrusions by the same pathogen.
- Our immune system is as unique as our fingerprints and there are many dietary, lifestyle and genetic components which affect its uniqueness.
- The male and female immune systems vary greatly and it's believed that the hormones oestrogen and progesterone, along with the genetic composition of females, contribute to the female immune system generally being stronger than males'.

- The immune system plays an important role in mediating allergies, which are not to be confused with food intolerances.
- A poor diet can contribute to an increased risk of obesity and nutritional deficiencies. This may result in inflammation and an increased risk of some chronic diseases.
- We should aim to support our immune system, rather than 'boost' it.

CHAPTER 3

The Role of the Gut on Immune Function

What Is the Gut?

In Chapter 2 we explored the barriers involved in the immune system, with the gut being one of the key barriers. Aside from its role in immunity, the gut has recently become the latest hot topic in the conversation about health. Scientists have discovered that it may be as influential to our health as the brain. Unfortunately, as a result of the rise in interest around gut health, there has simultaneously been an increase in the number of myths associated with the gut. The gut is commonly mistaken for the stomach and, while both are vital components of digestion, they are in fact very different organs.

The gut is the 9-metre-long digestive tract, which begins in the mouth and runs through the body to the colon. However, when you hear people refer to gut health, typically they are referring to the gut microbiome: a collection of bacteria, fungi and viruses located inside the large intestine. The gut microbiome is rather sizeable and accounts for around 3 per cent of our total body weight.

A deeper understanding of the capabilities of these microbes has only really come about in the last twenty years, thanks to advances in clinical nutrition research. As encouraging as this is, the research is still very much in its infancy and we have a whole lot more to learn about the gut and the role of the microbiome. That said, we are aware that these microbes are far more power-ful than we initially gave them credit for – we actually have more microbes than we do genes or skin cells. So, technically, we're comprised of more bacteria than anything else. It's understood that the gut can influence multiple areas of our physiologi-cal function and everyday wellbeing, including our hormone function, sleep, dietary preferences, energy absorption and uti-lisation, weight management, blood glucose regulation, mental wellbeing, neurological health, and of course it plays a critical role in the immune system. The gut microbiome is also able to support the production of some vitamins such as vitamin B1 (thiamine), vitamin B7 (biotin) and vitamin K2. Consequently, it's evident why the gut is commonly referred to as the second brain. It really does have a colossal influence over our wellbeing, therefore optimising it and nourishing it in the best way we can is essential for promoting optimal health and immune function.

How Does the Gut Affect the Immune System?

With over 70 per cent of our immune cells located in the gut, it's no wonder that the gut plays such a pivotal role in supporting optimal immune health. Many of the immune cells in the gut are the components of the adaptive immune system. Since the internal lining of the gut is only one cell thick, it's considered to be a vulnerable site of infection. This may help to explain why so many of the immune cells are housed in the gut – to ensure they're ready to fight when necessary.

Supporting a healthy gut lining is central to protecting the immune function. When the integrity of the gut lining is compromised the microbiome bacteria can easily penetrate the lining and pass into the bloodstream. Even the commensal types of bacteria (these are the good, or beneficial, bacteria that help to support our general wellbeing) can be problematic should they seep into other areas outside of the gut. Thus they can still trigger an immune response, contributing to unnecessary and undesirable inflammation. If this occurs regularly there is a greater risk of chronic inflammation and inflammatory-related diseases.

The integrity of the gut lining can be compromised via a variety of dietary and lifestyle factors including:

- **High intakes of fructose** Fructose is a sugar which is most well known for its presence in fruit. Nowadays, it can be extracted from fruit and used as a 'healthier' sugar in many food products. A common example of this is agave syrup, which is regularly used in place of sugar and honey. However, compared to consuming fructose contained within a whole fruit, isolated fructose is far more problematic for the gut lining. This is because when fructose is consumed as part of a whole fruit, the fibre in the fruit is also being consumed. It is the fibre which helps to protect the gut lining and can work to counteract some of the problematic impacts of the isolated fructose. It is worth noting here therefore that the presence of fructose in fruit is not a valid reason to exclude fruit in the diet. Rather than focusing on the fructose in the fruit in your diet, try to be mindful of consuming isolated fructose without the presence of fibre, for example in syrups such as agave, products which use fructose as a sweetener, or fruit juice in excess.

- **High intakes of saturated fats** Saturated fats are also known to disrupt the integrity of the gut lining. Saturated fats are commonly found in fried foods and ultra-processed foods such as fast food, sweets, chocolate bars, cakes and biscuits. Where possible, try to limit these in the diet due to their damaging effects on the gut.

- **Overuse of non-steroidal anti-inflammatory drugs (NSAIDs)** NSAIDs are typically used to manage pain and inflammation and include common medications such as aspirin, paracetamol and ibuprofen. Many NSAIDs are over-the-counter drugs, while others require prescriptions. The abuse of NSAIDs has been shown to cause damage to the gut lining. While there are of course circumstances where the use of NSAIDs is required to manage pain and inflammation – and they are deemed very safe to use – they needn't always be the first port of call. Where possible, try to utilise other dietary and lifestyle protocols first (where safe to do so), either instead of or alongside the use of NSAIDs.

- **Overexposure to environmental toxins** Environmental toxins are practically impossible to avoid. We're constantly exposed to pollution via transport, toxins in our foods and skincare, perfumes and cosmetic products, air fresheners, candles, room sprays, household cleaning products, furniture, clothing, plastic containers, food packaging and so much more. While you may not be able to avoid them entirely in your day-to-day life, you may want to consider opting for products with more natural ingredients. Reviewing your regular cleaning products and cosmetics and replacing them for more natural alternatives can be a great way to limit your exposure to environmental toxins.

Supporting the Gut Lining

There are multiple dietary and lifestyle factors and habits which can positively or negatively influence the integrity of the gut lining. While some may be out of our control, making small changes where possible can help promote the strength and reduce the permeability of the intestinal lining. Becoming more aware of the influences outlined next is a great place to start.

Limit exposure to unwanted external pollution

This is no easy task and may seem quite daunting; however, asking yourself the following questions can help it to feel that bit more achievable. Can you seek fresh air where possible? Do you have access to green space in which you could spend 5–10 minutes per day? Could you consider investing in a water filter to reduce toxins in your everyday drinking water? Water filters are available in all variations nowadays and while you can have them installed into your water systems, water filter jugs can be really effective too. Additionally, becoming more aware of food packaging and limiting the number of food products you buy that are wrapped in plastic can help to reduce your exposure.

Limit alcohol use

The overconsumption of alcohol can also contribute to the impairment of the gut lining. Alcohol and the by-products of alcohol metabolism have been shown to contribute to inflammation in the gut. High levels of inflammation caused by alcohol can cause damage to vital organs, specifically the liver, which in turn impairs the ability to effectively metabolise alcohol and thus further contributes to inflammation, resulting in a vicious cycle. High levels of inflammation in the gut can also increase the permeability of the gut lining and therefore compromise its integrity. Where possible try to opt for three or four alcohol-free days per week and limit your total consumption to no more than the maximum recommended intake of fourteen units per week.

Limit the use of unnecessary medications

It's so easy to reach for a painkiller as a precautionary measure. However, try to ensure you're only using non-steroid anti-inflammatory drugs (NSAIDs) when really necessary and if you think an ice pack or a heat pack might calm your headache or period pain then try these first. Examples of NSAIDs include over-the-counter pain relief medications such as aspirin and ibuprofen.

Eat mindfully

Eating mindfully can have hugely powerful health benefits. Living in a more mindful manner is steadily becoming more widely practised, although, the truth is, many of us aren't fully clued up on what it really means, why it's important or even how to practise it. Eating mindfully is arguably one of the most important things you can do for your health. Let me explain.

The very first phase of digestion is known as the cephalic phase, and it is initiated before food even enters your mouth. During this phase, the brain engages with the thought that you're expecting to receive food. It is activated in this way via sight and smell, our environment and feelings around food. Once it's acknowledged that food is going to be arriving soon, the brain sends chemical messages via the vagus nerve to the stomach, where hydrochloric acid and the digestive enzymes pepsin, gastrin and histamine are secreted in readiness to break down the food particles upon their arrival. Once the food has been broken down in the stomach and turned into what is known as chyme it can pass into the small intestine and then into the large intestine, where the nutrients can be absorbed and the fibres used to feed the beneficial bacteria in the gut.

Now imagine an all-too-common scenario: you're eating while you're doing your emails or having a meeting. Your brain is fully engaged in the emails or the content of the meeting you're in and consequently it's not stimulating the first stage of digestion, the cephalic phase. As a result, your brain hasn't had a chance to send the messages to the stomach alerting it to expect your food. The stomach is then ill-prepared and has to work harder and faster once the food arrives. In turn, the food often isn't fully broken down, meaning that larger particles of partially digested food can end up entering the gut. This can cause disruption to the gut as it's unable to utilise these larger food particles which can contribute to impaired gut function and an increased risk of intestinal permeability. This can often be experienced through symptoms such as flatulence and bloating. Eating more mindfully can really help to support nutrient absorption as the food can be adequately broken down, ensuring that the nutrients can be absorbed through the gut lining and into the blood. What's more, the primary satiety hormone leptin, which sends a signal to your brain indicating that you are full, will be secreted faster when the cephalic phase of digestion is fully engaged. As a result, you'll be fuller and more satisfied from the food you're eating.

Simple ways to eat more mindfully include:

1. **Eating slowly.** This can be challenging initially and slightly uncomfortable so try putting your cutlery down between each mouthful. This will also encourage you to chew your food more, which makes it easier for the stomach to break down. It's generally recommended that we chew each mouthful twenty times – although this may sound excessive, it's a useful guideline to promote increased chewing.

2. **Avoiding distractions.** Distractions such as scrolling on your phone, responding to emails, reading articles or watching TV can turn your brain's focus away from the food and towards the activity you're engaged in. Where possible, remove tech from the table and set a rule to make time for lunch during your working day, to allow for optimal digestion.

3. **Engaging in the process of eating.** As the cephalic phase of digestion begins before we even taste our food, it's really important that we try to involve our brain with the thoughts, smells and visual aspects of our food.

Mindful eating can be awkward and definitely requires a degree of initial commitment and practice, so rather than trying to change your eating behaviours overnight start by focusing on mindfully eating one snack a day. Once you've got to grips with this you can move on to your main meals, although bear in mind that this may not always be possible with every meal; for example, when you are eating in the company of others. Of course, there are many other benefits of eating with people, particularly for our social wellbeing, so there is no need to practise mindful eating to the detriment of your time with others. However, if we can remove the habits associated with our tech and eating that's an excellent place to start.

What Is the Role of Short-Chain Fatty Acids (SCFAs) in Gut Health?

Our gut microbes predominantly feed off fibre in our diets. Fibres are indigestible types of carbohydrate and they are one of the main components of our diet that allow our gut bacteria to survive and thrive. The process of feeding the gut microbiome generates by-products known as short-chain fatty acids (SCFAs). These SCFAs are incredibly powerful and beneficial products which can be used by the body in numerous ways.

The most common types of SCFAs are acetate, butyrate and propionate. These are metabolites (a by-product of metabolism), which can be transported around the body in the blood and are associated with a wide range of beneficial health effects. They also fulfil a multitude of roles, including regulating blood glucose levels, managing the absorption of energy from our food and supporting the production and function of T-reg cells. T-reg cells are the cells that decipher when to switch the T-cells (discussed in the previous chapter) on and off; they can also manage anti-inflammatory mechanisms when required. Another main role of SCFAs is to send chemical messages to the brain from the gut via the vagus nerve. This is the long nerve which runs through the body from the brain into the gut.

SCFAs also provide a source of fuel for the immune cells located in the gut. More specifically, butyrate provides around 70 per cent of the energy that is required to support the cells located in the intestines. These cells are important for promoting adequate nutrient absorption from food.

Potentially even more interestingly, SCFAs have been shown to reduce the power and virulence of pathogenic bacteria that may invade the body, which is another way they can help to protect us and improve immune function. Furthermore, along the gut lining we have small junctions of cells known as tight junctions; this is where the cells come together to support the barrier so it's important that these remain intact in order to help maintain the strength of the gut lining. SCFAs can help to protect the tight junctions from unwanted damage, allowing them to continue to support the gut lining.

What Does a Healthy Gut Look Like?

Understanding what gut health means is an excellent place to start, but identifying a healthy gut can be surprisingly challenging.

The gut can house thousands of different types of bacteria at any given time and, generally speaking, these bacteria typically fall into two camps: the commensal bacteria, otherwise known as the 'good' or friendly bacteria, and the pathogenic bacteria, commonly known as the 'bad' or less beneficial bacteria. A healthy gut is one that has a well-balanced microbial profile. That does not mean an *even* balance – it should contain more commensal than pathogenic bacteria but still maintain a fine equilibrium between the two. Typically, the greater the area which the beneficial bacteria populate in our gut, the less room there is for pathogenic bacterial species. The question is, what is an unbalanced gut microbiome and what are the signs? An unbalanced gut is one which has some of the following:

- Too high levels of either friendly or unfriendly bacteria (neither is great).
- Bacteria which is present in the small intestine (we want it to live within the large intestine).
- Poor microbial diversity.
- Low levels of bacteria overall.

It can be useful to think of the gut as a garden. When we plant pretty flowers and plants we need to ensure they're provided with the necessary nutrients to survive, such as light, soil and water. If we neglect the plants, they'll die off, which can leave a larger area in the garden for weeds to grow. Over time, if this continues, our garden will have a far higher percentage of weeds than attractive flowers. If we liken the gorgeous flowers and plants to the beneficial bacteria in the gut and the weeds to the pathogenic bacteria then we can start to see how important it is for us to maintain healthy habits and consume a nutritious diet. This allows the beneficial bacteria to grow, thrive and survive. In later chapters I'll highlight the key dietary and lifestyle habits we can adopt in order to nourish our gut and the microbes within it.

There's a common misconception that poor gut health will only be presented via gut-related symptoms such as bloating, flatulence, pain, discomfort or changes to bowel movements. In fact, symptoms of poor gut health can extend far beyond these typical symptoms and can also include brain fog; difficulty concentrating and performing optimally at work; poor sleep; changes to your skin; weight gain; fatigue; mood disorders such as depression or anxiety; nutrient deficiencies and of course an impaired immune function and heightened susceptibility to illness.

Having said this, many of these ailments are multifactorial so while the gut can be related to these symptoms, the presentation of these symptoms alone doesn't necessarily indicate poor gut health. Should you be concerned about any gut-related symptoms it's always advisable to seek personalised advice from your healthcare provider.

Supporting a Healthy Gut Microbiome

In response to the influx of new discoveries about the gut, the gut health industry has exploded in recent years. As a consequence, more and more people are now aware of the impact of gut health. Unfortunately, this has also led to thousands of products making wild claims of unsubstantiated health benefits. While there are certainly some products that are valid and beneficial, it is not always the best approach to go straight to advertised products. There are some simple dietary steps you can take to optimise your gut microbiome without burning a hole in your wallet.

Eat more fibre

Fibre really is the fuel which feeds our beneficial gut bacteria. It's what they feed off and ferment in order to produce those beneficial short-chain fatty acids (SCFAs). Fibre also helps to promote healthy bowel movements as it contributes to increasing stool bulk and transit time, which is particularly important for those who struggle with constipation.

There are two main types of fibre: soluble and insoluble. Soluble fibre feeds the beneficial bacteria and encourages the production of SCFAs, as mentioned above. Additionally, it helps to absorb water in the intestines which creates gel-like substances comprised of waste products. These substances can pass through the gastrointestinal (GI) tract more easily and can contribute to softening the stools. Soluble fibre is particularly important for those who struggle with diarrhoea or constipation as it encourages bowel movements and absorbs excess water in the stools. Soluble fibre also plays a role in slowing down the release of sugars from your food into the bloodstream and therefore can be important in managing blood glucose control.

As a result of these qualities, it also increases satiety, keeping you fuller for longer. Soluble fibre can be found in wholegrains, oats, milled flaxseeds, chia seeds, beans and pulses.

Conversely, insoluble fibre provides more roughage, which is needed to increase stool bulk. It's commonly found in the skins of fruits and vegetables, nuts and seeds. However, many plant foods will contain a combination of both soluble and insoluble fibre. As a result, rather than focusing on the types of fibre you're consuming it's more important to focus on the variety of sources of fibre.

Aiming for thirty different types of plants each week is a really sound way of incorporating a range of fibres and increasing diversity in the diet. This may sound daunting at first but considering that every fruit, vegetable, lentil, pulse, wholegrain, herb and spice you consume accounts for one type of plant you'll quickly see that it is far more achievable than it sounds. As an example, consider a vegetable and chickpea curry made using courgettes, onions, leeks, peppers, spinach, chickpeas, garlic, cumin, paprika, coriander, black pepper and chilli pepper. Serve this with brown rice and you've hit thirteen different plants in one meal. Are you up for the challenge?

Limit antibiotic use

This may appear to be a controversial recommendation; even more so when I along with many others owe our lives to antibiotics. In my case, if my immune system hadn't responded to the multiple courses of antibiotics I was subject to as a result of an MRSA infection, I wouldn't be writing this book!

It goes without saying that there are of course circumstances when we need antibiotics in order to survive. However, they are definitely still being given out far too readily. Despite the pushback from many healthcare professionals and doctors to reduce the use of antibiotics and protect against antibiotic resistance, it appears that they're still often being prescribed as a precautionary measure. Since antibiotics do not distinguish between beneficial bacteria and the targeted unwanted pathogen, their impact is often to significantly reduce the number and diversity of *all* the bacteria in the gut. While this has the desirable outcome of removing the unwanted bacteria, it can simultaneously threaten our beneficial bacteria too. In the aftermath of a course of antibiotics, it can be a race for time as to whether the commensal or pathogenic bacteria can populate the gut microbiome fastest. Which side wins is often dependent on our dietary and lifestyle behaviours.

Incorporate more fermented foods and drinks into your diet

Fermented foods are foods which have been left to grow live cultures. They contain a variety of bacteria and bioactive compounds, which, when they reach the gut, can help to colonise the commensal bacteria. For this reason they have been strongly associated with more beneficial gut microbial profiles and a multitude of health benefits. Fermented foods are not new to our society; in fact, they've been consumed for thousands of years. It's only recently that they've become more 'on trend'.

Fermented foods have been shown to help support our immunity as they can increase our resistance to unwanted bacteria and infections. As a result, they should be something which we try to incorporate into our daily or weekly diet. Yoghurt is an excellent example of a fermented food; however, where possible, opt for unflavoured and unsweetened options and look for those containing live cultures in the ingredients list. Unfortunately, not all yoghurt contains live cultures these days. Much like yoghurt, kefir, a fermented milk drink, can also be a smart way to populate the gut with live cultures. The same rules apply so try to look for live cultures on the ingredients list.

Miso, sauerkraut, kimchi and kombucha are all also popular sources of fermented foods and drinks. Miso is a Japanese paste made from fermented soya beans, which can be mixed with warm water to make soup or incorporated into vegetable dishes and dressings. It also provides that delicious umami flavour to really add taste to your food. Sauerkraut and kimchi are fermented vegetable dishes that are excellent for incorporating into salads or adding to sandwiches or wraps to provide an extra hit of live cultures with your lunch.

Finally, kombucha, a fermented tea drink, can be a useful alternative to alcoholic drinks or sugar-sweetened beverages. The production of kombucha has been highly commercialised, meaning some kombucha products can be very high in sugar and contain no live cultures so always read the labels whenever you can.

Unfortunately, with the increase in popularity of fermented foods, many commercial fermented foods undergo processing methods to help speed up fermentation. Such short cuts often don't allow the live cultures to fully cultivate. Additionally, other popular processing mechanisms such as smoking, baking or pasteurising can destroy the beneficial bacteria in fermented foods. Therefore, try to source genuine fermented foods where you can or try to make your own, which can be easy to do and far more economical.

Integrate prebiotic-rich foods into your diet

Prebiotic fibres are a type of fibre which help to feed the beneficial bacteria in the gut. Think of them as the soil, water or light which are essential to nurturing the plants in your garden. Prebiotic-rich foods may also help with supporting the intestinal barrier by encouraging mucus growth around the gut lining, and have been found to help manage blood sugar regulation and moderate appetite. Prebiotic fibres can be found naturally in a whole host of foods including garlic, green bananas (the less ripe the banana, the more prebiotics it contains), leeks, chickpeas, Jerusalem artichokes, apples, inulin (which is now being used in some products to create a slightly sweeter taste) and chicory root. Adding these foods to your diet regularly can help to encourage the growth and survival of the beneficial microbes.

Pack in the polyphenols

Polyphenols are chemicals which are found naturally in plants and have been shown to be beneficial in supporting the immune function and promoting a healthy gut environment. The rate of absorption from polyphenols can vary greatly and can often be dependent on factors related to the gut, such as the microbes and the digestive enzymes already present, along with the chemical structure of the food or drink in which the polyphenols are found.

Polyphenols are metabolised in the gut and throughout the metabolism process by-products known as metabolites are created. These metabolites may be even more bioavailable than the polyphenols themselves, meaning that the metabolites created from the metabolism of the polyphenols may be able to be absorbed and utilised more efficiently than the polyphenols. It's these metabolites which have been associated with anti-inflammatory, antimicrobial and anti-allergic effects. Since the relationship between polyphenol absorption and metabolism and the gut is bidirectional, it's important that we consume a variety of polyphenols in the diet alongside utilising other dietary and lifestyle tools to promote a healthier gut microbiome where we can. Polyphenols can be found in a variety of plant foods, including fruits, vegetables, seeds, herbs, coffee, cocoa, tea and wine (yes really, but all in moderation!).

Focus on your water intake

Water plays an essential role in moderating the digestive system and ensuring your bowels are moving regularly and efficiently. Water is absorbed in the large intestine, the site where food is converted into solid stools, so when fluid consumption is particularly low, the lack of water can contribute to harder stools that are more difficult and uncomfortable to pass. These types of stools may also have an increased transit time, which can contribute to alterations to the gut microbiome.

The recommendation is to consume around two litres of fluids per day. However, excess heat and increased exercise or sweating will mean that you need to increase your intake. Where possible try to listen to your body and drink to thirst. You should also be mindful that consuming too much water can be detrimental to maintaining fluid balance and the dangers of its effects can often be underestimated. Assessing the colour of your urine is a useful tool for managing your hydration status: dark urine that has a smell to it can be indicative of dehydration. Where possible, aim for a light yellow to clear colour. However, be aware that some supplements, such as those containing B-vitamins, can make urine appear a fluorescent colour and some foods such as beetroot may also alter its colour. If you're at all concerned about the colour of your urine or your hydration status always seek advice from your healthcare professional.

Limit the use of sweeteners

Artificial sweeteners, or non-nutritive sweeteners, are calorie-free ingredients which are often added to foods to increase their sweetness or palatability. They are significantly sweeter than sugar and are often used in commercial food products to provide the sweetness that consumers crave without the perceived impact on blood glucose levels, or the calories that are found in sugar. However, recent research questions the impact that they may have on blood glucose control, and some studies suggest they may contribute to impaired blood glucose regulation. It's also noteworthy that they can alter and drive the desire for sweetness that many people have. Instead of replacing one with the other, we would benefit from limiting our sugar *and* sweetener intake. Although artificial sweeteners have previously been deemed safe there are now rising concerns around their long-term health implications due to the quantities in which we're consuming them. Artificial sweeteners are consumed in a whole range of products on a daily basis and since 2018, when the UK introduced the sugar tax, the use of artificial sweeteners has increased dramatically. They are commonly found in low-calorie and sugar-free or 'no added sugar' foods and drinks spanning a range of categories including flavoured fizzy drinks, flavoured milks and waters, protein bars and powders, squash, cereal bars, yoghurts, chocolate bars and more.

Some artificial sweeteners can contribute to impaired gut symptoms when consumed in excess, resulting in cramping, bloating and even laxative effects. Some studies have shown that they may also have the ability to alter the intestinal bacteria. However, we do require further research on humans to confirm this but, in the meantime, it is recommended to limit them in your diet where possible.

Avoid using mouthwash

On the surface, mouthwash appears to be a rather harmless and, if anything, beneficial addition to our oral hygiene routine. However, some emerging evidence suggests that the use of a chlorhexidine mouthwash (antibacterial mouthwashes) can contribute to lowering the abundance and the diversity of the bacteria in the gut microbiome. While we do need more research, limiting your use of antibacterial mouthwash may help to contribute to improving your gut health. Although do ensure you continue with a good oral hygiene routine by brushing and flossing regularly.

I hope that you now have a wider understanding of the role of the gut on our overall health – and more specifically the immune system. Since such a significant number of immune cells are located in the gut, it stands to reason that in order to optimise our immunity it's vital that we focus on gut health. However, it's not solely the bacteria in the gut that we need to consider, we also need to factor in the impact of our dietary and lifestyle choices on the gut lining. The good news is that small changes such as increasing your plant consumption, fibre intake and fluid intake and reducing the overconsumption of saturated fats, alcohol and artificial sweeteners can have powerful benefits for your gut health.

In the next chapter we're focusing on the early years and how the foundations of a healthy gut can be laid from such a young age. Consequently, we can start to form a full picture of the complex relationship between the immune system, the gut, our environment and the body as a whole.

Summary Points

- With 70 per cent of the immune cells located inside the gut, supporting a healthy gut environment is pivotal to optimising immunity.
- The gut microbiome consists of a range of bacteria, viruses and fungi located in the large intestine.

- The gut can house thousands of different types of microbes at any given time. These microbes can be commensal (beneficial) or pathogenic (less beneficial).
- A healthy microbiome is one which is well balanced between the commensal and pathogenic bacteria.
- Fibre ferments to feed the beneficial bacteria. The fermentation process produces short-chain fatty acids as a by-product. SCFAs have a wide range of benefits including supporting the integrity of the gut lining, promoting T-cell regulation and modulating the effects of the unfriendly bacteria.
- You can support your gut microbiome by incorporating more fibre, plant-rich foods and fermented foods into your diet and consuming adequate amounts of water to stay hydrated.
- Limiting antibiotic and NSAID use, artificial sweeteners and saturated fats in the diet can help to support a healthy gut.

CHAPTER 4

The Early Years

I now want to draw your attention to the early years of life. The influence of the early years on health and the immune system is not something that is always acknowledged, so you might be surprised to hear that this is actually one of the most critical periods of life. In this chapter I'll walk you through why this stage is so important and how we can best support children growing up under our care.

It's at this time where both the gut and the immune system undergo major developments in response to the environment. We are all born with an immature immune system which can increase the susceptibility to infections and disease. However, laying the foundations for supporting a healthy gut and a healthy immune system is pivotal during these early years.

This chapter is more relevant to parents or prospective parents and caregivers and therefore if this feels less relatable or applicable feel free to skim past it to Chapter 5.

The Role of the First Thousand Days of Life

Contrary to what this may imply, the first thousand days of life is actually defined as the period from conception and the time spent in utero up until the child's second birthday. This has been shown to be the most critical time in the development of the cognitive, emotional and physical health of the child and is fundamental to nourishing and nurturing a healthy gut microbiome and a well-functioning immune system. Additionally, it is a period of rapid development for the metabolic, hormonal, neuronal and endocrine pathways and evidence has suggested that disruptions during this phase can impact the physical health outcomes (including immunity) later on in life. For the baby, the first thousand days poses a significant, heightened susceptibility to environmental influences. As a result, if an infant is exposed to high levels of stress in the early years, they're at a greater risk of developing a less resilient stress response later on in life. These changes can contribute to long-term adverse effects on physical health, immune health and mental wellbeing later on in life.

As a result, the behaviours of parents, guardians or caregivers can substantially impact a child's future health outcomes. For example, the use of recreational drugs or an overconsumption of alcohol by caregivers – and even the economic circumstances in which the child has grown up – can all influence their health at a later stage.

However, this is not to say that a child's health outcomes and immune function are completely pre-determined by their parents or caregivers. They are contributing factors to the bigger picture. It's important that we have an understanding of this, because even though we can't change the circumstances into which we were born, we may be able to influence prospective parents or those caregivers looking after young children.

Since we've just explored the importance of the role of the gut microbiome on the immune system, I don't need to reiterate how crucial it is to nourish a healthy gut. The first thousand days of life are an indispensable time for building the foundations of a healthy microbiome, laying the groundwork for an optimal immune function and setting the stage for later on in life. Protection, nourishment and support during this phase is key to increasing the chances of supporting a beneficial gut microbiome for the long term.

Within the first thousand days there are three primary stages of laying down the foundations of a healthy gut and promoting the development of a healthy immune system.

1. Conception

There are, of course, numerous circumstances where diet and lifestyle do not influence the ability to conceive, and for many individuals and couples, conception isn't straightforward. There are many contributing factors that affect fertility, a number of which can be manipulated or corrected through dietary and behaviour changes. For example, the microbiome of both the male and the female can play a contributing role in the ability to conceive. In addition to the gut microbiome, the vaginal microbiome can also markedly affect conception outcomes. In some cases when the vaginal microbiome is imbalanced, the immune system can drive up inflammation. In turn, this may impair the ability of the sperm to swim to meet the egg.

Furthermore, the endometrial lining and the sperm contain their own microbes, and the types of microbes contained within these components can also alter fertility success rates. Consequently, if both the male and female focus on optimising their gut microbiome and immune health during this time, they may be able to increase the chances of conception. Evidence now also shows that the health and nutritional status of both parents at the point of conception can influence the health of their offspring too. Therefore, if you're prospective parents, you may want to think about optimising your health ahead of trying to conceive.

2. Pregnancy

During pregnancy, maternal health is undoubtedly the greatest contributor to the health and development of the foetus and their immune system. The relationship between the maternal immune system and that of the foetus is a bidirectional one. Early on, the mother's immune system adapts to accept the foetus and the placenta, but if this adaptation doesn't occur, the mother's immune system is at risk of rejecting the foetus or the placenta.

In response to this adaptation, the immune system has to work harder throughout the whole pregnancy as it is required to protect both the mother and the foetus against harmful pathogens. As a result, the immune system of the mother is often compromised throughout this time. This can explain why a pregnant woman may be more susceptible to cold and flu viruses than they otherwise would be.

In utero the foetus's immune system can be challenged by external and internal environmental exposures to pathogens and high levels of stress. In response to these challenges, the mother's immune system is able to pass antibodies through the placenta to the foetus to help protect and strengthen their immunity. As antibodies can be passed through to the foetus, evidence shows that the foetus can often develop a tolerance towards maternal vaccinations in utero too. While this doesn't protect the offspring entirely, it can increase their tolerance and reduce their susceptibility to specific pathogens in the early days of life. Consequently, this can also help to set up their immune system for the later years.

Conversely, high levels of maternal stress throughout pregnancy can impair immune development and increase the risk of adverse health outcomes later on in life. Furthermore, chronic low-level inflammation or infections in the mother or in the placenta have been associated with an increased risk of growth deficits, disease and allergies in the offspring. Evidently managing stress and exposure to pathogens where possible can help to support the foetus's immune development.

It should come as no surprise that maternal nutrition throughout this period plays a critical role. Throughout pregnancy the mother's nutrients are required to support not only her own immune system but the development of the foetus's: as a result, her nutritional requirements increase. Those looking to conceive, as well as pregnant women, should focus on ensuring they are reaching the necessary intakes for the nutrients required to support the growth of a foetus.

Iron, folate, iodine, vitamin D and zinc have been highlighted specifically as key nutrients required to support immune health in the mother and the offspring throughout pregnancy. Furthermore, these nutrients will also be playing multiple other roles in the body in order to support the mother's normal physiological function and the growth and development of the offspring. During this time the mother should also focus on general health and nutrition advice as this will also be relevant for supporting their own health and immunity.

While we are still incredibly far off identifying the exact

mechanisms which are impacted by internal and external factors in utero, pregnant women and those of childbearing age can use this information to optimise their diets and lifestyles in the best way they can.

3. The first two years of life

How a baby is born is not always something that is in the control of the mother and therefore while the mode of delivery can impact the development of the offspring's microbiome, it's not always controllable and there are many other dietary and lifestyle behaviours which can support the offspring's development of a healthy gut microbiome. However, where there is a choice between a vaginal birth and a Caesarean delivery, it's useful to have the relevant information to help you make a decision.

Evidence demonstrates that babies born vaginally have microbiomes similar to the mother's birth canal and babies born via a Caesarean delivery display microbial profiles similar to the mother's skin. Vaginally born babies tend to have a more diverse microbiome following their delivery when compared to those born via C-section. Although, remember, the delivery method alone does not solely determine the outcome for the offspring's microbiome.

The first two years of life are hugely influential in the development of the offspring's health and immunity as there are many other means of helping to promote a healthy gut microbiome independent of the delivery method.

As soon as a baby enters the world, the environment starts to shape their gut microbiome. There are hundreds of contributing factors which can positively or negatively affect gut health: the home environment, food consumption, pet exposure, experiences with farmyard animals, medications and products used inside and outside the home environment can all assist in moulding the microbiome and the immune system. (Many of these factors I discuss in more detail later on.)

Research has demonstrated a link between non-communicable diseases (i.e. those which cannot be passed through a contagious infection) that occur later on in life and dysbiosis in the gut during childhood. Furthermore, research conducted in low- to middle-income countries has shown that there is an association between exposure to enteropathogens (the unwanted pathogens which are carried through soil, food and water) in the early years and an increased risk of diarrhoea and infections. These enteropathogens can contribute to an increased risk of systemic inflammation, inflammation in the gut and impaired growth later on in life. These examples go to show how influential these early years can be and how, although we may not always be able to identify the impact of our exposures straight away, they can have long-lasting effects.

It's important to note that although the first thousand days make a weighty contribution to setting up a positive microbial environment and more optimal immune system, what we do throughout our life can positively or negatively alter both the microbiome and the immune system.

Nutrition in the First Two Years

As we've seen, the first thousand days are critical in promoting a healthy gut profile, which in turn can help to support the development of healthy immune systems, both innate and adaptive. Beyond this period, appropriate nutrition and environmental exposures in the first two years of life can also positively influence immune function.

These first few years can be a great way to lay the foundations for forming healthy habits and attitudes towards nutrition and lifestyle, ones that the child can carry throughout their childhood and into adolescence. Although we are focusing specifically on the first two years, we shouldn't ignore the role of the rest of the childhood and adolescent periods will have on the immune system's development.

Breastfeeding

There are many factors which contribute to whether or not a baby is breastfed and it's vital that we aren't elevating one feeding method over another as all fed babies are well-fed babies. Nutrition and health are not the only areas of consideration when it comes to feeding your baby. Factors such as maternal ability, mental wellbeing, socio-economic status, education, baby's responsiveness, religious beliefs, personal beliefs and confidence all play a major role in whether or not a baby is breastfed. Every mother, father or caregiver who feeds their children with love and care is doing a phenomenal job.

However, as a nutritionist it's my role to present the research and recommend accordingly. With that in mind, and from a purely nutritional standpoint, there are some benefits associated with breastfeeding. While the quality of breastmilk is affected by the maternal diet, generally speaking breastmilk contains a wide variety of bioavailable nutrients, which are required for the general growth and the development of the immune system. (The bioavailability of a nutrient refers to how much of it can be absorbed and utilised in the body.)

These nutrients include the fat-soluble vitamins A, D, E and K, the water-soluble vitamins B and C, and the minerals calcium, iodine, iron, magnesium, phosphorus and many more. Additionally, breastmilk also contains enzymes which are required for the development of the immune cells and immunoglobulins, a type of antibody which helps to support the ripening of the immune system and fights against unwanted disease and infections. The amino acids and long-chain fatty acids present in breastmilk also help to promote a healthy immune function.

Additionally, breastmilk contains human milk oligosaccharides. These are a type of carbohydrate which have prebiotic properties and can help to positively cultivate the gut microbiome. The quantity and quality of human milk oligosaccharides found in breast milk can vary greatly depending on environmental and genetic factors.

Evidence has shown that the majority of the bacteria within the microbiomes of breastfed babies in the first six months are predominantly derived from human milk oligosaccharides. This is particularly beneficial for the baby's health and immune system as it helps to cultivate a gut profile rich in beneficial bacteria. These bacteria are able to produce the short-chain fatty acids (SCFAs) which we discussed in Chapter 3. The beneficial bacteria and the production of SCFAs can help to promote a healthier environment for the immune cells to function in.

Furthermore, the beneficial bacteria 'infant-type' bifidobacteria has been found to be one of the most dominant types of bacteria in a breastfed infant's gut. Infant-type bifidobacteria are those which are more likely to colonise in an infant's gut compared to an adult's microbiome. Although bifidobacteria are beneficial bacteria for both infants and adults, infant-type bifidobacteria has been associated with an enhanced immune development and lower levels of intestinal inflammation. This type of bifidobacteria may also play a role in the production of short-chain fatty acids, which are associated with reducing intestinal permeability and supporting the production of mucus and the integrity of the tight junctions. (Tight junctions play a role in preventing permeability of the gut lining.) These benefits can often be just as achievable in formula-fed babies since many baby formula milks now contain fructo-oligosaccharides and galacto-oligosaccharides, which can also contribute to increasing infant-type bifidobacteria and have been associated with a reduction in atopic disease risk. One randomised control trial provided 134 infants with a combination supplement of the prebiotic fibres fructo-oligosaccharides and galacto-oligosaccharides or a placebo for the first six months of life. The results showed that those infants on the prebiotic supplement showed a significantly reduced risk of atopic dermatitis, recurrent wheezing and allergic urticaria in the first two years of life when compared to the placebo group. The researchers suggested that the mechanism behind these benefits is down to the manipulation of the gut microbiome.

The types of microbes present in the gut in the early years have also been shown to affect the risk of allergic diseases later on in life, and inappropriate colonisation of pathogenic (or less beneficial) bacteria may increase the risk of conditions such as asthma and eczema. However, higher levels of the beneficial bacteria (infant-type bifidobacteria) in the early years have been associated with a lower risk of these conditions.

In today's modern world, we're fortunate to have access to some high-quality formula milks which are able to support all your child's nutritional needs in order to encourage healthy growth and development. Furthermore, appropriate baby pre- and probiotics can also help to support the development of the gut microbiome.

Always seek advice from your midwife or healthcare provider before considering supplements for your child, or if you're unclear how best to support your child's nutritional requirements.

The role of weaning and beyond

Weaning is the process of introducing a child to foods beyond their usual breastmilk or formula milk. My weaning days were very much an enjoyable experience (so I'm told) and while not every child begins with the same love and enthusiasm for food, this is the perfect time to introduce those positive emotions and experiences towards mealtimes and food in general.

The recommended age to start the weaning process is around six months. However, this will vary between babies, as some will show signs of readiness slightly earlier and others marginally later. The weaning process can be an ideal time to introduce babies to a wide range of food groups containing varying tastes, textures and visual components. The more diverse the range of foods that a child is introduced to at an early age, the more likely they are to enjoy a wide variety of foods later on in life. Consequently, this can be a really important time to help establish a healthy balanced diet for your child.

Research has shown that the mother's diet during pregnancy can also influence taste preferences. Children born to mothers with a sweeter taste preference throughout pregnancy are likely to have sweeter palates. Similarly, mothers who consume bitter greens throughout the second and third trimesters can increase the likelihood of their offspring eating bitter green vegetables such as spinach and broccoli.

Incorporating a variety of whole foods into the diet throughout the weaning process can introduce the child's gut microbiome to the beneficial effects of different types of fibres and plant chemicals such as polyphenols. Incorporating a range of nutrients into the diet at this stage is pivotal for priming immune cell development, as undernutrition can contribute to impaired immune health in later years, so regularly offering diverse ingredients and new foods is vital in conditioning the immune system. It is commonplace for babies to reject certain foods, but by continually exposing them to these foods in a variety of forms and combinations you will increase the likelihood that they'll grow to enjoy a variety of foods. Where possible, don't avoid certain foods simply because your baby has rejected them once. Additionally, allowing your infant to watch you eat can also help to encourage them to explore new foods and flavours. Where possible, try to lead by example and act as their role model to help to stimulate them to develop a positive relationship with food.

The introduction of solid foods is the first time that a baby may be exposed to new antigens from food, which can both challenge and strengthen their immune cells. Understandably for many parents, the weaning stage can be intimidating and nerve-racking due to potential allergen exposures. However, evidence suggests that early exposure to potential allergens may help to reduce the risk of developing an allergy later on in life. Potential allergens should always be given separately to other foods and in small amounts to begin with. These potential allergens include cow's milk, eggs, foods containing gluten, nuts and peanuts, seeds, soya, shellfish and fish. If you're particularly nervous or anxious about offering allergens, you can always offer these within the safety of a hospital environment or in a location which is relatively close to a healthcare practice. For more safe weaning advice please seek advice from the NHS website. Remember, weaning can be a stressful experience for some parents, so focusing on creating a relaxed environment can be really helpful; that way you will be supporting your baby's metabolism, the development of their gut microbiome, nutrient absorption and their immune system.

It's fascinating to see how the immune cells begin to become primed so early on and how the foundations for a healthy gut can be laid from such a young age. Those first thousand days, from pre-conception throughout pregnancy and into the first two years, can really set the child up for a healthier life later on. For prospective parents, current parents or caregivers it's incredibly exciting and empowering to know that the food you feed your children from a very young age can influence them in later life.

As busy parents or caregivers, sometimes life can feel a little overwhelming and not every aspect of your child's birth or early years may be in your control – just remember you're doing your best and that's the most important aspect of being a parent or caregiver.

As adults we can't do anything to change the environment in which we were brought up. However, remember that it's never too late to make positive changes to your diet and lifestyle. In the next chapter, I'm going to focus more on the specific nutrients we require to support our immunity – these can, of course, be introduced at any age!

Summary Points

- The first thousand days of life is a crucial period in the cognitive, emotional and physical development of a child. It's this period which helps to lay the foundations for a healthier immune system and gut later on in life.

- The maternal and paternal health at the point of conception and the mother's diet throughout pregnancy can significantly influence the offspring's health and immune system later on in life.
- Exposure to external pathogens and vaccines in pregnancy can contribute to increasing immune tolerance in the offspring.
- The first thousand days are a critical period for developing a healthy gut microbiome, which is a key part of the foundations for promoting a healthy immune system. However, habitual diet and lifestyle changes can be made throughout life which can positively or negatively impact the gut microbiome and the function of the immune system.
- Factors such as delivery method, method of feeding, exposure to pets, environmental factors and economic status can all impact a child's health outcomes and their immune function later on in life.
- Human milk oligosaccharides found in breastmilk provide rich contributions to the development of a healthy immune system and gut microbiome in the early years.
- Weaning and the introduction to solid whole foods is a perfect opportunity for increasing diversity of the gut microbiome and supporting adequate nutritional intake.

CHAPTER 5

The Role of Macronutrients and Micronutrients on Immunity

While we may not be able to turn back time to influence our early years, one thing we can do is focus on the foods we're consuming today, tomorrow, next week, next month and so on.

In this chapter we'll be diving into nutrition on a deeper level and the roles of macro and micronutrients, which sit at the very heart of nutrition. In Chapter 1, I introduced the definition of nutrition as 'the process of providing or obtaining the food necessary for health and growth'. Macro and micronutrients are the nutrients which are contained within the foods necessary for health and growth. Every food contains at least one of the macronutrients. The health-promoting foods are rich in a wide range of micronutrients. These nutrients contribute to supporting the roles of the immune cells. Think of them as the fuel that allows the cells to carry out their necessary jobs. You've likely heard the analogy which suggests you wouldn't put diesel into a petrol car and expect it to work efficiently. In the same way, we can't expect the immune system, the gut or any other aspect of the body to work optimally without adequate fuel.

Additionally, nutrition isn't merely about what we are consuming, it's also about what we're *not* consuming. For example, following a restrictive diet, whether it's driven by ethical or religious beliefs, taste preferences or pre-conceived ideas about nutrition, may contribute to an increased risk of deficiencies if we are not compensating with micronutrients from other sources. Those living in a food secure environment are often eating a minimum of three times per day and it's the decisions that we make on a constant basis which can help or hinder our short-term and long-term health. Therefore, ensuring we're consuming a wide range of adequate nutrients is imperative to supporting immunity and health in general.

In this chapter, I'm going to break down the fundamentals of nutrition and dig into the roles that the macro and micronutrients play on supporting our immune system.

What Are Macronutrients?

The macronutrients in our food constitute the foundations of nutrition and they play a vital role in supporting our body to carry out its wide range of complex duties every day. Macronutrients are those nutrients which are required in large amounts daily. Most people will be able to name three types of macronutrients: proteins, fats and carbohydrates. However, there is, in fact, a fourth: water. Water is essential for the body to function so thinking of it as the fourth macronutrient is particularly important as so many of us are not consuming enough water each day.

Calories and why they matter

A calorie is the amount of heat which is required to raise one gram of water by one degree Celsius. Consequently, calories are the unit used to quantify the amount of energy in a food or drink. Calories are essential to maintaining life as the energy delivered via our food and drink enables us to carry out normal physiological functions such as growth, respiration, metabolism, blood circulation, hormone production and, of course, supporting our immune cell function.

Not all macronutrients contain the same amount of calories per gram. Carbohydrates and proteins provide four calories per gram while fats contain nine calories per gram. However, it's important to note that not all calories are utilised equally. Calorie requirements also vary greatly between individuals and are dependent on a variety of factors including age, height, sex, activity levels, muscle mass and lifestyle habits.

As a society we're rather calorie obsessed and although managing a healthy balance with regard to calorie intake is necessary, it's not quite as simple as solely focusing on calories. It's true that chronic overconsumption of calories can increase the risk of obesity and have a negative influence on systemic inflammation and the immune system. Conversely, a chronic underconsumption of calories can also have detrimental effects on immune health.

As we'll explore further, *where* we get our calories from is vital in supporting immune function and managing inflammation. Not all calories are derived from equal sources and the macro and micronutrients in our food play an undeniably fundamental role in supporting immunity too. For example, 100 calories from oats are not equal to 100 calories from sweets. The oats contain fibre, which reduces the total amount of calories absorbed from the oats, whereas the calories in sweets come predominantly from sugar and will have a much higher absorption rate. Additionally, oats contain a variety of micronutrients such as iron and B-vitamins to help support the immune function, whereas the sweets contain little nutritional benefit.

Calorie restriction – what you should know

Striking the balance between energy intake vs energy expenditure is important when we're thinking about calories in general. Some research suggests that moderate calorie restriction may have some beneficial effects on the immune system. By moderate calorie restriction, I'm referring to a minor reduction in calorie intake, although still ensuring adequate amounts of energy intake to prevent malnutrition. Malnutrition is commonly depicted by an image of someone with a very low body weight but it's important to understand that it can also manifest in healthy weight or overweight individuals who are not consuming adequate amounts of macro or micronutrients.

Moderate calorie restriction has been shown to be beneficial in supporting immunity. One study found that an average of a 14 per cent calorie restriction in individuals aged between twenty-five and forty-five contributed to improving immune health. The results showed an increase in the size of the thymus gland, which plays a role in the production of T-cells. Consequently, this led to an increase in the number of T-cells produced when compared to the control group on their normal calorie intake.

The calorie-restricted group also presented a downregulation of a specific gene known as Pla2g7, which plays a role in driving an inflammatory response. To fully understand the implications of this reduction of Pla2g7, the researchers then bred mice without this gene and assessed the impacts on their metabolic and immune health. The findings suggested that these mice were less likely to gain weight on a high-fat diet and had a reduced risk of fatty liver disease, inflammatory markers and an increase in the size and efficiency of the thymus.

This evidence suggests that moderate calorie restriction may play a role in supporting immune health in some individuals. By the same token, it's important we consider the role that calorie restriction has in these outcomes. It's arguable that the outcomes caused by the calorie restriction may have been due to a reduction in high-sugar, high-fat foods rather than the calories themselves. While this looks interesting, we're not yet at the stage of suggesting that calorie restriction independent of diet quality can induce this response.

In addition, research has explored the effects of moderate calorie restrictions on the gut microbiome. Evidence suggests that the adaptations to the gut microbiome in response to moderate calorie restriction may contribute to improvements in immune function and a delay in the development of chronic inflammatory diseases.

However, the long-term implications of calorie restriction on immune cell function are not yet fully understood as we don't yet have enough long-term studies in this area. Furthermore, as we age, we should consider the negative implications of calorie restriction. These can include an increased risk of nutrient deficiencies, impaired mental wellbeing and energy malnutrition. Additionally, severe calorie restriction (above 40 per cent restriction) can induce detrimental adverse effects to the immune system.

So, calories aside, let's now look at each of the macronutrients in turn.

Carbohydrates: friend or foe?

Carbohydrates often receive bad press. However, they are key to our general health and for supporting energy production. They are the body's preferred source of fuel and are one of the most abundant sources of energy in our food. Carbohydrates are broken down into glucose and then used to make ATP (adenosine triphosphate), which is the body's usable source of energy. Glucose which is not used instantly is converted into glycogen and stored in the muscles for use later on.

Carbohydrates are divided into two main categories based on the size of their molecules: simple carbohydrates and complex carbohydrates. The benefits of each vary greatly. However, they're often classified in unison and demonised equally. Simple carbohydrates are faster-releasing and play an important role in producing energy quickly. This is particularly helpful during sporting events where we might need a quick energy hit. Typically, they have a low satiety value and can spike blood sugar levels instantaneously. Examples of simple carbohydrates include fruit juice, syrups, honey and sweets to name a few. On a day-to-day basis, simple carbohydrates are the ones we should aim to limit in the diet.

Complex carbohydrates contain dietary fibres (a type of indigestible carbohydrate), which slow down the release of the sugars into the bloodstream and increase satiety. Examples of complex carbohydrates include beans, pulses, wholegrains, fruit and vegetables.

When it comes to supporting the immune system, carbohydrates are pivotal due to their role in generating energy. When the immune system is under attack it has to work extra hard to fight off intruders. It is required to send additional chemical messages, create new immune cells and generate antibodies. These are all tasks that demand a lot of energy. As a result, carbohydrates are vital for supporting these energy requirements.

Carbohydrates should make up around 45–50 per cent of our total energy intake. That said, where possible try focusing on complex carbohydrates as this is a great way to increase fibre intake too. I'll discuss fibre and the key role it plays on immune health in more detail later.

Try these tips for incorporating more complex carbohydrates into the diet:

- Switch your morning high-sugar granola or muesli for lower sugar options.
- Opt for brown rice over white rice.
- Change your white pasta for wholegrain pasta.
- Switch biscuits and cookies for oatcakes with hummus.
- Try adding more starchy vegetables to your meals, such as sweet potatoes, butternut squash, parsnips and carrots. Where possible, try to keep the skins on as this can be a great source of fibre.

- Incorporate beans and pulses to bulk out mince-based recipes.

Protein: essential for growth

Dietary protein sources are made up of individual amino acids. Protein is most well known for its role in muscle growth and repair. Protein also plays a vital part in hormone production, cell structure, cell regeneration and metabolism.

Dietary protein sources are broken down into individual amino acids in the body and utilised accordingly. The amino acids are sub-grouped into three categories:

1. Essential amino acids – we cannot create these in the body and therefore they must be consumed through the diet.
2. Non-essential amino acids – we can produce these in the body and therefore it's not imperative that we consume them through the diet.
3. Conditionally essential amino acids – these can be made by the body in small amounts or under certain conditions. Trauma, pregnancy and illness are some examples where the demands for the conditionally essential amino acids outweigh how much the body makes. Therefore we must obtain the short-fall through our diet.

Typically, animal sources of protein (meat, fish, eggs and dairy) are considered complete proteins. This means they contain all of the essential amino acids. It can be more challenging to find complete protein sources from plant foods but quinoa, soya products, buckwheat and hemp are all considered to be complete protein sources. Consequently, in response to the rise in veganism and plant-based diets, diet diversity (particularly of plant-rich protein sources) is imperative as this can help to ensure you're getting a range of amino acids and therefore reduce the risk of specific amino acid deficiencies.

It's common to believe that we are not getting enough protein, as we are constantly being marketed more and more high-protein products, from snack bars, to sports drink and protein powders. In reality, the majority of people are getting ample amounts of protein. In the UK the recommendations are to consume 0.8–1g of protein per kilogram of body weight: for example, a 70kg individual would require between 56 and 70g of protein per day. Although, those who are particularly active may benefit from slightly higher intakes. Furthermore, athletes will also require significantly greater intakes.

To provide some context, a medium-sized egg contains 6g of protein, one tablespoon of peanut butter provides around 4g of protein and 100g of chicken breast contains around 28g.

When consumed alongside carbohydrates, protein slows down the release of the carbohydrates into the bloodstream. This can help to support sustained energy and satiety. Protein also has a higher thermic effect, meaning that it requires more energy to metabolise than carbohydrates or fats. This further contributes to increased satiety from protein. As a result, consuming a source of protein at each meal and snack can help to keep you fuller for longer.

Protein is one of the most important macronutrients in supporting immune function as each of the individual amino acids have relevant roles within the immune system. These roles include the activation of B-cells and T-cells, production of natural killer cells and macrophages, the multiplication of lymphocytes, gene expression and the production of antibodies and cytokines. Essentially, they have a leading role in supporting many of the mechanisms within the immune system. In the rare cases in which amino acid deficiencies may occur, it may be necessary to supplement with specific amino acids in order to support immunity and reduce the risk of illness and disease. (See Chapter 10 for more on supplements and always seek advice from your GP or healthcare professional.)

Fats: the good, the bad and the ugly

Fats are the densest source of dietary energy as they contain 9 kilocalories per gram. As a result, there's a very common misconception that consuming dietary fat simply contributes to weight gain. In response to this thinking, the low-fat movement grew exponentially and it's only been in more recent years that we're slowly starting to understand that some fats have a crucial role in supporting our overall health, wellbeing and immune function. Their roles include promoting the absorption of fat-soluble nutrients (such as vitamins A, D, E and K) and supporting heart health, membrane structure, hormone production and brain cell function.

There are three main categories of fats:

1. **Unsaturated fats** are known as the 'good fats' as they're the ones which contribute to our normal physiological functions outlined above.
2. **Saturated fats** are often found in ultra-processed foods and are well known to raise low-density lipoproteins (the bad cholesterol).

3. **Trans fats** have been shown to increase low-density lipoproteins and decrease high-density lipoproteins (also known as good cholesterol), a combination that is considered to be the most harmful to our health. Trans fats are also found in ultra-processed foods and can be produced as a result of frying foods and heating unstable oils to very high temperatures.

Fats are also critical in supporting the immune system as they're key for developing the structural components of cell membranes, they play a vital part in mediating inflammation and they're the precursor for eicosanoids. Eicosanoids are molecules which send signals around the body to gather more help when the immune cells are under attack. The aim is to focus on consuming unsaturated fats in our diet. These are found in foods such as avocados, nuts, seeds, olives and olive oil and oily fish such as salmon, mackerel and sardines. The recommendations are that fats should make up around 20–35 per cent of our total dietary intake.

Omega-3 fats

Omega-3 is a nutrient which is often associated with brain health. Omega-3 is a type of polyunsaturated fat and is particularly noteworthy when it comes to immune function. Omega-3 fats are sub-grouped into long-chain and short-chain fatty acids. The long-chain fatty acids – eicosapentaenoic acid (EPA) and docosahexaenoic acid (DHA) – are the active forms of omega-3, which can be utilised in this form in the body. Typically, EPA and DHA are found in animal sources such as oily fish, particularly salmon, mackerel, sardines, anchovies and herring, although DHA can also be found in algae sources.

The short-chain fatty acid alpha-linolenic acid (ALA) needs to undergo a conversion process into EPA and DHA in the body before it can be fully utilised. Throughout the conversion process we lose some of the ALA, therefore the quantity of active omega-3 from ALA is lower when compared to EPA and DHA. ALA is found in plant sources such as walnuts, flaxseeds, seaweed and chia seeds. Due to the limited dietary sources and poor conversion rates, obtaining adequate amounts from plant foods can be challenging. Therefore, those on a vegan diet may need to consider a high-quality supplement.

Omega-3 and its role in the immune system has been a focus of much scientific research for many years and consequently its role in supporting immune health is well understood. Omega-3 exerts beneficial effects on both the innate and the adaptive immune cells. When omega-3 is metabolised it produces metabolites which help with reducing inflammation in the body. Metabolites are by-products which are produced naturally through metabolism. It's these anti-inflammatory effects that give omega-3 its 'anti-inflammatory' status. Let me explain how these anti-inflammatory effects work.

Omega-3 predominantly affects the neutrophil, macrophage and dendritic cells (all types of white blood cells) in the innate immune system. The white blood cells are the cells which race to the site of infection first. Omega-3 can help to reduce migration of the neutrophils, which means they're more likely to stay at the primary site of infection in order to carry out their roles. In other words, once the neutrophils are at the site of attack omega-3 can encourage them to remain at the site in order to fully carry out their job. Omega-3 has also been shown to increase phagocytosis, the process whereby the neutrophil ingests or kills the intruder. Omega-3 can also help to suppress the activity of the dendritic cells once they have completed their job of highlighting the intruding pathogens to the T-cells.

Furthermore, omega-3 positively influences T-cells and B-cells within the adaptive immune system as it helps to reduce the activity of the T-cells and B-cells once they have completed their operation. Additionally, it can downregulate cytokines and increase T-regulatory cells to promote the desired anti-inflammatory effect following an immune attack.

Omega-6 is another common omega which is often very much misunderstood, particularly in relation to the immune system. Omega-6 can be found in nuts, seeds and seed oils, although it is more prominent in higher-sugar, higher-salt foods and ultra-processed snacks such as biscuits, cake bars, crisps and processed meats.

While it is true that the roles of omega-6 are more proinflammatory, acute inflammation isn't always quite as detrimental as it's made out to be and omega-6 plays a very vital role in immunity. As we explored in Chapter 2, the ability to generate an inflammatory response is actually a key part of a successful and healthy immune system. Omega-6 helps to produce the proinflammatory mediators which encourage the immune cells to attack the unwanted pathogens. Omega-6 is commonly found in dietary sources in the form of linoleic acid. Linoleic acid is converted into the active form, arachidonic acid, in the body. It's this molecule which is able to send the proinflammatory messages in order to increase inflammation at the site of infection.

Rather than demonising omega-6 altogether, it's more important that we focus on obtaining a healthy omega-3 to omega-6 ratio. Since omega-3 and omega-6 compete for the same pathways in order to be utilised, having too much omega-6 could result in a more chronic proinflammatory environment.

Typically, the western diet is much higher (and arguably far too high) in omega-6 fats since they're far more abundant in high-fat, ultra-processed foods. In order to improve your ratio of omega-3 to omega-6, try to incorporate two portions of fish per week into your diet (oily if possible), add flaxseed to your breakfast and try switching your ultra-processed snacks for a handful of walnuts. Additionally, you may benefit from limiting ultra-processed foods and vegetables oils where you can. Since we do need some omega-6 in the diet, nuts, seeds, tofu and eggs can be great ways to obtain adequate amounts.

Stay hydrated

Water is the fourth but equally essential macronutrient that is required to maintain everyday physiological function. Water's main roles include transporting nutrients around the body, carrying waste products to the kidneys for filtration and excretion, maintaining homeostasis, supporting digestion, maintaining moisture in the skin, providing a lubricant for our joints and supporting fluid production. Staying hydrated is also important for maintaining blood pressure.

Dehydration (or hypohydration) occurs when we're not consuming enough fluid to support our physiological demands. Just 1–2 per cent dehydration can contribute to a dry mouth, fatigue, headaches, irritability, confusion and even reduced cognitive function. Consequently, even slight dehydration can strongly impair your daily performance.

In severe cases, there can be detrimental effects from dehydration. One study showed that dehydration following a judo practice caused a reduction in immune cell function and white blood cell function. Ensuring that we're staying hydrated is crucial for supporting not only our general physiological function but ensuring that the immune system can work optimally too.

Additionally, it's not uncommon to mistake thirst signals for hunger signals when you're dehydrated. I'm sure we've all experienced a time where we thought we were hungry and opted for a snack, which didn't fill us up, so we've had another snack and then a glass of water, only to realise that we were in fact just thirsty in the first place. Consequently, consistent dehydration may also contribute to increased calorie intake.

The risk of dehydration can be higher in certain groups and in particular circumstances. For example, babies and infants, who are unable to monitor their own fluid balance; the elderly, who may be less aware of their fluid intakes or the signs of dehydration; athletes who experience excessive sweating during extreme heat and the average individual when we simply don't consume enough fluid throughout the day.

Below are some top tips to help you increase your water consumption:

- Try carrying a water bottle with you everywhere you go. Nowadays there are water stations everywhere which you can use to fill up on the go.
- Set reminders on your phone throughout the day. A notification can be a great way to remind you to drink.
- Try adding herbs or fresh fruit to your water bottle as this can increase the palatability of the water and may make you more likely to want to drink it.

What About Micronutrients?

Micronutrients are nutrients which are required in much smaller amounts than macronutrients but are no less important. They are required to support normal everyday physiological function and consist of vitamins and minerals. Vitamins are vital amines, meaning that with a few exceptions (namely some B-vitamins and vitamins D and K) they can't be produced by the body and must be consumed through the diet. Minerals are naturally occurring chemical elements that are required to support our physiological function.

Vitamins

There are two main types of vitamins: fat-soluble and water-soluble vitamins. Fat-soluble vitamins can be stored, and reserves are kept in the liver, muscles and tissues, whereas water-soluble vitamins cannot be stored in the body and must be consumed almost daily to obtain adequate status. There are six categories of vitamins, all of which play varying roles in supporting immune function.

Vitamin A

Vitamin A can be found in two main forms: provitamin A and preformed vitamin A. Provitamin A is the precursor to vitamin A, meaning that in order to be utilised it must undergo a conversion process. However, preformed vitamin A can be utilised in its natural form.

Provitamin A is usually found in the form of carotenes. Carotenes need to be converted into preformed vitamin A in the body in order to be utilised. As a result, carotenes have a lower bioavailability than preformed vitamin A. This means less of the vitamin A from carotenes can be absorbed and utilised as some of it is lost through the conversion process. Since carotenes are found in a wide variety of foods (largely plant foods but also eggs and dairy) we don't necessarily need to consume more preformed vitamin A to account for the losses. Carotenes have antioxidant capabilities, which means they can stabilise the otherwise unstable free radicals. Free radicals are molecules which can contribute to oxidative stress, cell damage and cell death. Carotenes can be found in many plant foods such as green leafy vegetables, carrots, sweet potato, butternut squash, tomatoes, eggs and dairy.

Preformed vitamin A can be used in its current state and can also be found in eggs and dairy products and liver. Liver is well known for being the most abundant source of preformed vitamin A.

Along with its antioxidant capabilities, vitamin A has also been shown to help with the growth and regulation of many of the immune cells.

The B-vitamins

B-vitamins are a group of water-soluble vitamins that are needed for multiple regulatory and metabolic mechanisms in the body. These include energy metabolism, protein synthesis and DNA production. The immune system is taxing on our energy levels and therefore ensuring we have adequate intakes of the B-vitamins can help with optimising energy levels to support immune function. In addition to their general roles, there are some B-vitamins which execute more specialised roles within the immune system.

While it is believed that some B-vitamins can be synthesised in a healthy gut, they can't be generated in the quantities in which we require them and therefore it's important we consume them through the diet. Additionally, the synthesis of B-vitamins in the gut may rely on ensuring that the gut is in an optimal condition to be able to produce these nutrients. The requirements for intakes vary between the different types of B-vitamins due to their stability, bioavailability and roles in the body. Despite B-vitamins being relatively abundant in our foods, our modern-day lifestyles can increase the risk of deficiencies in certain cases. Factors such as high levels of stress, the use of drugs and alcohol and consuming vegan or plant-heavy diets can increase the need for B-vitamins. Additionally, these needs can also heighten during pregnancy and illness.

- **Vitamin B6 (pyridoxine)** The chemical name for vitamin B6 is pyridoxine and its specific roles include aiding the production of lymphocytes and interleukin-2 (IL2). IL2 is a type of cytokine which sends signalling messages around the immune system. Vitamin B6 deficiency has been shown to decrease lymphocyte proliferation (i.e. the rapid reproduction of lymphocytes) and decrease antibody production. However, if you're consuming a varied healthy diet you should be eating adequate amounts of vitamin B6 as sources include fish, beef, eggs, liver, potatoes, bananas, cheese and nuts.
- **Vitamin B9 (folic acid or folate)** The dietary form of vitamin B9 is referred to as folate. However, the supplementary form is known as folic acid. Folic acid is required for the formation of DNA, protein metabolism and red blood cell production, all of which are vital in

supporting immune cell function. Folic acid requirements increase during pregnancy as it also plays a crucial role in the formation of the spinal cord and deficiency in pregnancy has been shown to increase the risk of spina bifida. Dietary sources of folate include green leafy vegetables, beans, peanuts, liver and eggs.

- **Vitamin B12 (cobalamin)** Along with vitamin B9, deficiencies in B12 have been shown to affect the production of nucleic acids (such as DNA and RNA), protein synthesis and can contribute to inhibiting activity of the immune cells. The symptoms of vitamin B12 deficiency include vitamin B12 deficiency anaemia, fatigue and muscle weakness, nerve damage, memory loss, the inability to concentrate and confusion. Vegan and plant-heavy diets can increase the risk of vitamin B12 deficiency since the main dietary sources are meat, fish, eggs and dairy. While fortified spreads, fortified plant milks and nutritional yeast can provide some vitamin B12, these foods are often not enough to meet the nutritional requirements for vitamin B12. Consequently, those following a plant-heavy or vegan diet should consider taking a vitamin B12 supplement.

Vitamin C

Vitamin C is a water-soluble nutrient and is the most well-known vitamin in relation to the immune system. Vitamin C really has had its fair share of media attention as it plays a multitude of roles in supporting immune health. Firstly, it has antioxidant capabilities, meaning that it can neutralise free radicals and reactive oxygen species (ROS). Free radicals and ROS are molecules which can contribute to oxidation and cell damage in the body. It also contributes to supporting a wide range of cellular mechanisms in both the innate and the adaptive immune systems. Vitamin C is essential for maintaining the health of the epithelial barrier of the skin. The epithelial barrier is one of our first lines of defence and is therefore particularly key when we're thinking about preventing the intrusion of unwanted pathogens. It can also contribute to increasing the activity of those cells which are capable of phago-cytosis (the process of catching and destroying the unwanted pathogen). With regard to the adaptive immune system, vitamin C is required in the production intake of the T-cells and B-cells and is necessary in promoting the removal and clear-up of dead or damaged immune cells.

Strong research links vitamin C deficiency with a weakened immune system and a greater risk of infection. Vitamin C is a relatively unstable nutrient, meaning it can be sensitive to oxygen exposure and heat. However, the good news is that since vitamin C is rather bountiful in fruits and vegetables, if you're consum-ing the recommended minimum intake of five portions of fruits and vegetables per day, with one portion being around 80g, then the chances are you'll be getting at least the recommended 40mg per day.

Vitamin D

In recent years, vitamin D has become an incredibly popular nutrient. You might be surprised to hear that vitamin D is tech-nically not a vitamin but rather a hormone. This is because we have the ability to synthesise it ourselves. Vitamin D is synthe-sised in response to sunlight exposure in the summer months. Interestingly, you can tell if the sun is in the correct location to synthesise vitamin D if your shadow is shorter than you are.

However, factors such as sunscreen, skin colour, dark clothing, sun position, body fat percentage and age can all impact your ability to synthesise vitamin D from the sun. Since we can't synthesise enough of it all year round (particularly in the UK) it's considered to be a vitamin. This means we need to consume it in dietary sources or through supplements.

The latest research from the UK's National Diet and Nutrition Survey in 2019 shows that on average adults (aged nineteen to sixty-four) in the UK are consuming just 5.4µg (54 per cent of the recommended intake) of vitamin D per day from a combination of dietary sources and supplements. Since vitamin D is very difficult to obtain from the diet alone, the UK recommendations are to supplement with 10µg per day during the winter months. Dietary sources of vitamin D include eggs, salmon, mushrooms, milk and fortified plant milks.

Vitamin D helps to promote the movement of T-cells, which encourages them to reach the site of infection. It also contributes to supporting the activity of the natural killer cells, production of antimicrobial materials and promoting the activity of regulatory T-cells (Tregs).

In addition to supporting immune function, it also plays a vital role in supporting heart health, bone health and mental wellbeing. Evidence has linked vitamin D deficiency to an increased risk of low mood.

Furthermore, vitamin D works closely with calcium and vitamin K2. Vitamin D supports the absorption of calcium and vitamin K aids the absorption and utilisation of vitamin D. Vitamin K2 is largely produced by the bacteria in the large intestine; however, it can be found in some dietary sources such as cheese, egg yolks, green leafy vegetables and natto (a Japanese fermented soya product).

Vitamin E

Vitamin E is another fat-soluble vitamin which can be stored in the tissues. Much like vitamins A and C it also has antioxidant capabilities. Vitamin E has been shown to help support the cell membranes and the regulation of natural killer cells and the T-cells and B-cells involved in the adaptive immune system.

The best sources of vitamin E include mango, papaya, avocado, olives, almonds and sunflower seeds. Consuming a varied diet with a selection of healthy fats should ensure you're getting adequate amounts of vitamin E through the diet.

Vitamin K

Vitamin K is also a fat-soluble nutrient that plays an important role in blood clotting. Blood clotting is particularly important in the immune system as it enable cuts and grazes to be sealed and repaired in the event of an open wound. This process helps to prevent further intruders entering the body.

Vitamin K is particularly important in supporting bone health, which, of course, is vital for longevity.

Vitamin K is best found in green leafy vegetables, some meat, cheese, eggs and natto (a fermented soya product).

Minerals

Similarly to vitamins, minerals are also essential in the diet. However, they're required in smaller amounts than the macronutrients. Interestingly, it's their chemical structure which differentiates them from vitamins. Vitamins are organic compounds while minerals are inorganic compounds. Minerals tend to come through the soil and work their way into plants and are much less vulnerable to heat and light than vitamins. They play a number of different roles in the body and ensuring you're consuming a variety of minerals through your diet is key to supporting an optimal immune function and general health and wellbeing.

Zinc

Zinc is a micronutrient that cannot be stored in the body and therefore we require a daily intake from dietary sources. It plays a key role in aiding immune function as it's required for cell growth and differentiation and immune cell signalling. It also helps to stabilise immune cell membranes, which can help to protect against oxidative stress. In addition to this, zinc is required in the production of pro- and anti-inflammatory cytokines and in wound healing.

Alongside its roles in immune function, zinc is crucial for general growth and development and supporting the integrity of the gut lining, which is paramount to a healthy immune system (see Chapter 3).

Zinc deficiency has been associated with a weakened immune system through its effects on both the innate and adaptive functions. Since zinc absorption decreases with age, older adults are at a greater risk of deficiency. In addition, gut disorders, overuse of drugs, alcohol and some medications along with restrictive diets can increase the risk of deficiencies.

Symptoms of a zinc deficiency include unexplained weight loss, changes to mood or appetite, hair loss and rough or very dry skin. If you're concerned that you may not be getting enough zinc in your diet it's recommended to seek advice from your healthcare professional. Although ensuring you're consuming a variety of meat and poultry, shellfish, nuts, legumes, wholegrains and fortified cereals will help to reduce the risk of deficiency.

Selenium

The quality of selenium in our food is heavily dependent on the quality of the soil in which the food is grown. Selenium has antioxidant capabilities and can therefore help to reduce free radicals and other reactive oxygen species that can contribute to oxidative stress and an impaired immune function. Additionally, selenium plays a role in the release of proinflammatory cytokines. Proinflammatory cytokines are particularly important for regulating the inflammatory response. Thankfully, selenium deficiency is rare in the UK.

Selenium is found in shellfish, Brazil nuts, liver, some grains and dairy products. Brazil nuts are particularly high in selenium and should therefore be consumed in moderation as overconsumption can pose a risk of selenium toxicity.

Iron

Iron is another familiar micronutrient with a vital role in immune function. It helps with supporting cell differentiation of the T-cells and B-cells in the adaptive immune system and also facilitates the generation of proteins and enzymes required to support immune cell function. Additionally, iron helps to transfer oxygen in the blood around the body. This is essential as the immune system requires ample amounts of oxygen to carry out its roles and fight unwanted pathogens.

Iron deficiency can impair the optimal function of the immune system so ensuring adequate levels is essential. Deficiency is common in female athletes, those following a vegetarian or vegan diet and women of menstruating age.

Iron is found in two forms: non-haem and haem iron. Non-haem iron is found in plant sources and has a lower bioavailability than haem iron which is present in animal sources.

Plant sources of non-haem iron include green leafy vegetables, oats, sesame seeds, lentils, quinoa and figs. Adding a source of vitamin C to plant sources of iron can help to increase the absorption. For example, try adding lemon juice to your spinach or broccoli or grate an apple into your porridge in the morning. Additionally, avoid consuming sources of non-haem iron with tea or coffee as the tannins in the tea and coffee can impair absorption. In practice, this means leaving around 45 minutes to an hour either side of your porridge in the morning before enjoying a tea or coffee.

Animal sources are the most bioavailable sources of haem iron and include red meat, offal, eggs and poultry.

Iodine

Iodine is a micronutrient that doesn't tend to get much attention in the media but nonetheless is one that plays a fundamental role in our health. It is a major component in optimising a healthy metabolism and growth and development. Furthermore, it's thought that iodine is important in helping to support a healthy balance between the proinflammatory and anti-inflammatory activities within the immune system.

Iodine is another nutrient which can be challenging to obtain on a plant-based diet as key sources include milk and white fish, although it can also be found in seaweed and algae, some fortified milk alternatives and prunes. If you follow a plant-based diet, I recommend checking the milk alternatives you're using as not all milk alternatives will be fortified with iodine. (Do also try to avoid milk alternatives with added sugars and syrups.)

Phytochemicals

Phytochemicals are compounds that are found naturally in

plants and have been shown to have a range of bioactive properties. They are widely recognised as supporting optimal gut health which, as we explored in Chapter 3, also plays an essential part in promoting a healthy immune system. Consequently, they are beneficial not only due to their anti-inflammatory and antioxidative properties but also indirectly through their influence on gut health.

Phytochemicals can be sub-grouped into a range of categories, all of which have slightly different benefits and are found in a range of diverse foods:

- **Flavonoids** These are a type of polyphenol and are one of the most well-researched groups of phytochemicals. They have been shown to help immune cell function by reducing inflammation via the modulation of the production of proinflammatory and anti-inflammatory cytokines. Flavanols (a type of flavonoid) can be found in foods such as apples, berries, grapes, tea, coffee and tofu.

- **Resveratrol** Most famous for its presence in red wine, research has shown that resveratrol may help counteract the development of inflammatory related chronic diseases such as diabetes, cardiovascular disease and neurological degeneration. However, it's important to highlight that studies of this nature often use very high doses of resveratrol in order to show a benefit, and consuming such high doses through diet is challenging – if not impossible. So while this research sounds promising, we cannot rely on resveratrol alone to manage the diseases mentioned above, although it is useful in highlighting the beneficial effects of resveratrol-rich foods in the diet. Resveratrol can be

found in red wine (drink in moderation), red grapes, peanuts, dried mulberries and rhubarb – to name just a few
sources.

- **ECGC** The scientific name for ECGC is Epigallocatechin-
  3-gallate. ECGC has significant antioxidative effects
  and can therefore help to fight free radicals and reactive
  oxygen species which, as a result, can help to reduce the
  risks of oxidation. Tea is a great source of ECGC with
  the concentrations being highest in green tea, although
  it's also present in oolong and black tea. Additionally, it
  can be found in fruits such as cherries, berries, apples
  and kiwi.

Incorporating a wide variety of plant foods into the diet can help
to optimise and diversify your polyphenol intake.

It's clear that macro and micronutrients carry out a wide
range of roles in order to support the immune system. To be able
to reach the recommendations and necessary requirements for
each nutrient, it is really important that we consume a variety
of foods as part of our daily diet. It's easy to fall into the trap
of eating the same foods day in day out for the sake of convenience. However, if you're not getting a wide enough range of
foods, there's an increased risk of nutritional deficiencies. All too
often we prioritise the macronutrients over the micronutrients. I
hope that this chapter has shown you that despite micronutrient
requirements being lower than those of macronutrients, they're
no less important for optimising immune health. Although I've
presented these nutrients predominantly in relation to their
roles in the immune system, it's important to remember that
they also play a multitude of roles in supporting many aspects
of our health.

In the next chapter we'll look in greater detail at how we can incorporate some of these nutrients into our diets. After all, we eat foods not nutrients!

Summary Points

- Macronutrients are those nutrients which are required in large amounts daily. While micronutrients are required in smaller amounts, they're no less important.
- Carbohydrates, proteins, fats and water are the four macronutrients, all of which have varying roles in the body.
- Obtaining a healthy ratio of omega-3 to omega-6 is crucial for managing proinflammatory and anti-inflammatory states.
- Vitamins and minerals all have individual roles that contribute to the health of the immune system.
- Phytochemicals are chemicals found naturally in plants and can provide extra support for the immune system.

CHAPTER 6

Incorporating Immune-friendly Foods into Your Diet

Now that you have a deeper awareness of how the immune system functions and some of the key nutrients responsible for upholding a healthy immune function, I want to focus on the practicalities of incorporating these nutrients into your diet. Ultimately, we eat foods not nutrients so it can be challenging to think about practical ways to incorporate these nutrients into a healthy balanced diet. As we've established from the start, I'm a firm believer that consuming a healthy diet needn't become another burden in an already demanding lifestyle. I'm going to show you that eating more immune-friendly foods won't necessarily require a complete overhaul of your current diet and that focusing on small tweaks can have a very positive overall effect.

In this chapter, I've picked out some key immune-friendly whole foods to incorporate into your diet, foods that can not only help to promote your immune function but can also support overall wellbeing. Ultimately, the benefits associated with eating more whole foods stretch far beyond immunity and can have a profound impact in other areas of our health, too. You'll also find recipes at the end of the book (see Chapter 11), which will provide you with some inspiration for incorporating these foods into your diet in a nutritious – but more importantly delicious – way.

Fruits and Vegetables

I'm sure it will come as no surprise to you that increasing the consumption of fruits and vegetables is key. Fruits and vegetables are abundant sources of vitamin C. Vitamin C is well recognised for its role in supporting the immune system and therefore fruits and vegetables can make a substantial contribution to supporting immune health. They are also packed full of a variety of fibre types to help nourish the beneficial microbes in the gut. Apples, pears, apricots and peaches are rich in pectin which is a type of prebiotic fibre that can encourage the growth of the good bacteria in the gut microbiome. Pectin has also been shown to have immunomodulatory effects on the production of cytokines. Additionally, some fruits and vegetables are rich in anthocyanins. Berries such as raspberries, blueberries, blackberries and strawberries are among those most abundant in anthocyanins. These plant compounds can have potent antioxidative effects so try to incorporate them into your diet on a daily or weekly basis.

Research has also shown that some fruits such as pomegranates contain a compound known as ellagic acid, which may have immunomodulatory effects and can contribute to the regulation of T-cell activity.

The research around the consumption of fruits and vegetables is extensive and it's clear that consuming more of them in our diet can help to support a whole host of positive health outcomes. A systematic review and meta-analysis of eighty-two studies highlighted a positive link between the consumption of fruits and vegetables and a reduction in inflammatory biomarkers. Additionally, the researchers concluded that regular fruit and vegetable consumption was positively correlated with a reduction in proinflammatory mediators and improved immune cell function.

In addition, another study conducted on eighty-three older individuals concluded that the consumption of five portions of fruits and vegetables per day increased their response to some vaccines, further highlighting the importance of continuing to consume fresh produce as we age.

The UK government recommendations are to incorporate a minimum of five portions of fruits and vegetables per day into the diet, with one portion being equivalent to 80g of fruits or vegetables. Given the nature of the food industry today there are many products making a dubious claim to be 'one of your five a day'. These include dried fruit products or dried fruit-based bars, juices and pasta sauces. However, in order to maximise the benefits of your five a day, where possible, try to choose whole fruits and vegetables as these will contain more of the fibres and beneficial nutrients that are often lost during the processing methods of many of these snacks and products. As we've already seen (see page 84), vitamin C is a moderately unstable nutrient, meaning it can be degraded by some of the processing methods. Frozen and tinned varieties do count towards your five a day. However, when you're opting for the tinned versions, pick those in water or natural juice rather than syrup.

Incorporating more fruits and vegetables into your diet can look as simple as:

- Adding mushrooms, tomatoes or spinach as a toast topper in the morning.
- Adding fresh or frozen berries to cereals or porridge for breakfast.
- Switching your glass of orange juice for a smoothie packed with frozen berries, spinach and kale (smoothies contain the whole fruit or vegetable including the fibre and therefore are a more fibre-rich option than juice).
- Incorporating spinach, sliced tomatoes or roasted vegetables into hummus and a falafel or chicken sandwich for lunch.
- Substituting white potatoes in mashed potato dishes for sweet potatoes, swede or turnips.
- Adding frozen spinach or sweetcorn to pasta dishes.
- Serving roasted vegetables alongside risotto or rice-based dinners.
- Blitzing cauliflower or broccoli into brown rice.

Beans and Pulses

It's not uncommon to feel indifferent to the idea of enjoying beans and pulses, also known as legumes. Despite the fact that they're more readily available than they have been in recent years, and more of us are eating them, many of us are still not familiar with how to prepare beans and pulses properly or how to really make the best of them.

Many people associate beans and pulses with a cup of dry, tasteless lentils which are presented after failing a bushtucker trial. However, with the right love, care and appreciation, beans and pulses can be the star of the show. It's worth making them the star because when it comes to immune function, beans and pulses are typically rich in protein, fibre and complex carbo-hydrates, all of which are essential in optimising immune cell health. Evidence has shown that the resistant starch present in these legumes can help to cultivate the beneficial microbes in the gut and support the production of short-chain fatty acids. Beans such as kidney beans, black beans and butter beans are rich sources of plant-based iron, magnesium and zinc.

Moreover, chickpeas, lentils, peas and beans are all affordable, accessible and versatile ingredients and the best part is that you don't have to be a chef to enjoy them properly. Tinned varieties can make incorporating them into any meal quick, easy and fuss free.

Try the following ideas for adding beans and pulses to your meals:

- Add lentils to mince-based dishes – not only will this increase the volume of your dishes and reduce the amount of meat used (and therefore the cost per portion), it will also increase fibre, complex carbohydrates and a whole host of micronutrient intakes.
- Blitz chickpeas or haricot beans into mashed potato or into soups.
- Use butter beans to make creamy pasta sauces.
- Add legumes to wraps and salads.
- Use kidney beans and black beans to make plant-based burgers.
- Roast chickpeas for a high-fibre, protein-rich snack. They are also a perfect alternative to nuts for those who are allergic. They can be added to soups and salads as a protein topper too.

It's important to note that drastically increasing the amount of beans and pulses in your diet within a short space of time can contribute to impaired gut symptoms due to the high fibre content. Therefore, rather than going from nought to sixty, slowly introduce a variety of beans and pulses into your diet and gradually increase the regularity and the quantity you're eating. Furthermore, soaking beans and pulses (or rinsing those from a tin) can help to remove some of the fermentable carbohydrates and may help ease the bloating and flatulence that can sometimes be experienced as a result of consuming beans and pulses. Soaking your legumes can also decrease the amount of phytic acid in them. Phytic acid can interrupt the absorption of some nutrients, although the benefits of consuming legumes far outweigh the negative aspects of phytic acid.

Nuts and Seeds

Nuts and seeds are nutritional powerhouses. They're loaded with a multitude of micronutrients and plant chemicals, which can be useful for topping up your levels to meet your nutritional requirements. However, nuts and seeds are typically high in energy and thus consuming them in moderation is recommended. Regular yet modest consumption can have significant beneficial health effects as they contain protein and healthy fats; more specifically, nuts such as walnuts are rich in ALA omega-3. Nuts also contain amino acids such as glutamine, which is essential for immune cell function, and micronutrients such as iron, magnesium, selenium, vitamin B6, vitamin E and zinc, all of which (as we saw in the previous chapter) support the normal and healthy functioning of the immune system. Incorporating nuts and seeds in your diet can be really simple.

Try the following tips for increasing your consumption:

- Sprinkle milled seeds onto yoghurt in the morning.
- Add nuts to salads or soups.
- Use soaked cashew nuts to make dressings or sauces.
- Incorporate walnuts and almonds into brownie or cake recipes.
- Switch your afternoon biscuits for a handful of mixed nuts.
- Blitz some Brazil nuts into your morning smoothie.
- Enjoy chia seed porridge for breakfast, an afternoon snack or dessert.

Cooking Oils

Cooking oils are currently a huge topic of controversy and confusion as there's so much misinformation around which oils we should be consuming and those that we should try to avoid or limit. The good news is that the beneficial cooking oils can contribute to our overall wellbeing and our immune system. On the flipside, if we overconsume ultra-processed oils with fewer benefits, then we could actually be contributing to higher intakes of omega-6 fatty acids, impaired immune function and increased inflammation. Thus it's important to be clear on which oils we should be consuming and why.

We are fortunate enough to have access to a vast range of oils, which are derived from a variety of plants such as nuts, seeds, fruits, vegetables and grains. Some oils are a source of monounsaturated fats and/or polyunsaturated fats while others, such as coconut oil, are much higher in saturated fats.

The health properties of oils are influenced by a number of factors. For example, the source and processing method of the oil has a dramatic effect on its quality and nutritional benefits, so consider the following questions when choosing oils:

1. **Is the oil from a single source or a blend of different plant oils?**
   Blended oils can often be of a lower quality; where possible try to ensure you're purchasing oils from a single source. Look on the back of the bottle, where it should provide information on its harvest. If it doesn't, then it may be that the oils are of a poorer quality. What's more, oils that have undergone significant processing are far more refined and consequently contain fewer beneficial compounds and vitamins. As a result, their flavour is often compromised. Unrefined or less refined oils are likely to be richer in flavour and contain far more nutritional benefits to support immune health.

2. **What is the smoke point of the oil?**
   The smoke point of an oil is the temperature at which the oil starts degrading, oxidising and releasing free radicals. This is particularly important as the oil can become rancid at the smoke point and may contribute to oxidation and an increase in free radicals in the body. This combination can cause damage to cells, particularly to the immune cells. Furthermore, when oils are heated beyond their smoke point they become unstable and can produce chemicals known as aldehydes. When consumed regularly and in excess aldehydes

can contribute to adverse health effects and may contribute to low-grade inflammation. The smoke points of each oil varies greatly: those which are typically considered to have higher smoke points include avocado oil, almond oil, olive oil and coconut oil to name a few. However, coconut oil is high in saturated fats and should therefore be used in moderation. There's a common trend where people have been adding coconut oil to their coffee, although this should be avoided due to the high saturated fat content. Coconut oil is better kept for use in Asian-inspired dishes where its aroma can really heighten the flavour of the dish. Conversely, avocado oil is one which we should be incorporating more into our diets and cooking, as it has a high smoke point but is less refined. It's also rich in key nutrients such as vitamin E and polyphenols.

3. **How is the oil stored?**

   The storage container of the oil can also affect its nutritional properties. For example, light can significantly contribute to degrading the bioactive compounds and nutrients in oils so they should be contained in dark bottles to protect them from overexposure to light. This is a useful way to identify the quality of the oil as those in clear bottles are likely to have been exposed to nutrient degradation in response to the light.

4. **In what dishes are you using the oil?**

   Some less refined oils typically have a lower smoke point and should therefore be used at lower temperatures or consumed raw in salad dressings and uncooked sauces in order to reap the full benefits. These include oils such as flaxseed oil, extra virgin olive oil, walnut oil and sesame oil. Flaxseed and walnut oils are rich in alpha-linolenic acid, a type of omega-3 which, when converted into the active forms of omega-3 in the body, can help to support the anti-inflammatory response. Unfortunately, unrefined oils are slightly more expensive than refined oils, so you'll probably want to consume them in moderation.

Which oils should we try to limit?

The use of vegetable oils has exploded over the past few decades as they've become one of the most mass-produced and cost-effective ingredients on the market. These are often made from a blend of vegetable oils that are high in omega-6. Furthermore, vegetable oils that are frequently used in commercial products are often hydrogenated vegetable oils. This means hydrogen has been added to the liquid oils in order to give them a more solid consistency and improve their shelf life. This process contributes to the development of trans fats, which are known to increase LDL cholesterol (the bad cholesterol) and decrease HDL cholesterol (the good cholesterol). An overconsumption of omega-6 fats and trans fats can contribute to an increase in low-grade systemic inflammation in the body.

In reality, consuming vegetable oils in the diet is rather unavoidable as they're used in so many food products and restaurant dishes. This brings us back to the point I made in the introduction, where I discussed striking a balance between your physical, mental and social health. You don't need to strive to entirely avoid oils, especially if it means you stop being able to enjoy certain foods and experiences. However, reducing them in your home cooking is a great place to start so, where you can, focus on olive oil and avocado oil for cooking and try to incorporate unrefined high-quality oils such as extra virgin olive oil, flaxseed oil and walnut oil into your salad dressings.

Wholegrains

Wholegrains have been a staple in our diets for thousands of years and it's only in more recent times that they've become overprocessed into cheap, less nutritious, more convenient versions known as refined grains. While there can be a place for refined grains within the diet, their role should be far more inconspicuous than it currently is. Because of modern-day overprocessing methods, grains are often miscategorised into less nutritious food groups. However, if we return to our roots and focus on *whole*grains, i.e. those that have not undergone overprocessing methods and remain intact, complete with the bran and germ, they can be highly valuable, nutritious components of our diet. One study compared the consumption of wholegrains with the consumption of white grains on an energy-matched western diet for a period of six weeks. Both groups were consuming the same amount of calories throughout the study. However, the sources of the calories differed. The research showed that those consuming the wholegrains demonstrated a significant increase in stool bulk, stool frequency and the presence of short-chain fatty acids, compared with those individuals consuming the refined grains. Additionally, the researchers found that levels of a proinflammatory bacteria species (Enterobacteriaceae) significantly declined in response to the wholegrain diet. This study goes to show how such a small change can make a considerable difference, even within a short time frame. Now imagine how powerful these small changes can be in your own body over the course of a few months, a year or even a few years.

Consuming wholegrains is often associated with consuming gluten-containing foods, which is not necessarily desirable or feasible for everyone. However, not all wholegrains contain gluten and those without gluten are just as nutritious and beneficial for our health. Gluten-containing wholegrains include wholegrain wheat, rye, barley and spelt, while non-gluten-containing wholegrains include oats, quinoa, buckwheat, amaranth, sorghum, teff and brown rice. Whether you're a gluten consumer or a gluten avoider there's definitely a case for incorporating more wholegrains into your diet.

Switching from refined grains to wholegrains is one of the simplest adjustments you can make in your diet and it can look like the following:

- Switching from white pasta to wholegrain pasta.
- Using brown rice instead of white rice.
- Reaching for wholegrain bread over white bread.
- Changing refined cereals for wholegrain varieties or a bowl of porridge.

Eggs

Up until the recent post-Covid rise in inflation in the UK, eggs were a cheap and accessible source of high-quality protein; even now they are a relatively cost-effective source of nutrients. Yet they have long been the topic of discussion and controversy. There are of course many justified environmental and ethical concerns around the consumption of eggs and animal products in general. While these concerns are absolutely valid and incredibly important, for now I am solely focusing on the nutritional content of eggs.

The myth around eggs being harmful to blood cholesterol levels began in the 1970s, but since then our scientific understanding and research capabilities have drastically improved. More recent research suggests that for the majority of individuals, eggs have little to no effect on low-density lipoprotein cholesterol (the bad cholesterol) but in some people they may increase high-density lipoprotein cholesterol (the good cholesterol) when consumed in moderation. In addition, eggs are rich in key nutrients such as choline, vitamin D, amino acids, selenium and zinc and consequently can be a nutritional powerhouse in supporting healthy immune cell function. Many of these nutrients are found within the yolks, so while egg-white omelettes are often hailed as the holy grail, you're far better off consuming the whole egg to obtain the maximum benefits.

As with all foods, eggs should be consumed in moderation and the general consensus is that two eggs per day is a safe and healthy target. Furthermore, if you are enjoying eggs in your diet try to ensure that you are buying and sourcing them as ethically as possible. In an ideal world we'd all be buying fresh eggs from the local farm, but we don't live in a perfect world so focus on doing the best you can. That may be buying your eggs direct from the local farm, opting for organic varieties or simply choosing the most ethically produced options you can afford. Our local food environment and resources will heavily impact the food we choose to purchase.

Meat and Fish

As with eggs, there are environmental and ethical questions to consider in the consumption of meat and fish. We all have a role to play in ensuring our food is sourced with care and concern for the environment and animals, but we needn't avoid them entirely in the diet – unless of course you have ethical or religious reasons for doing so. Meat and fish are complete proteins, meaning they contain all nine essential amino acids, and some of the nutrients present in meat and fish are more bioavailable than those found in plants. For example, iron bioavailability is significantly higher from meat and fish sources than from plant sources so if you're at risk of iron deficiency anaemia you may wish to consider increasing your consumption of animal sources.

Additionally, some nutrients such as vitamin B12 can be difficult to obtain from plant-based foods and therefore consuming meat and fish can help to optimise your intakes.

Furthermore, oily fish such as salmon, mackerel, sardines, anchovies and herring are all rich in omega-3, which helps to support the anti-inflammatory mechanisms within the immune system. It's recommended to aim for around two portions of fish per week, with one portion coming from oily fish, to ensure adequate omega-3 intakes.

Many of us are becoming more aware of the environmental impact of our diets and consuming less animal produce from more responsible sources can be a way of striking a balance between your health, your carbon footprint and animal welfare. Grass-fed, free-range, organic and wild produce may be more expensive but if you're replacing some of your animal proteins with plant-based sources you're unlikely to have to spend more on your diet overall.

Dairy

Sourcing ethically produced, high-quality dairy products is particularly important for supporting your immune health as it provides two key benefits. A good-quality dairy product is rich in vital nutrients such as healthy fats, proteins, calcium, phosphorus, vitamin D and iodine. Additionally, dairy is a source of live cultures. Choosing high-quality, unflavoured yoghurt and kefir containing live cultures is the perfect way to optimise a healthy diet and support immunity. Why opt for a strawberry-flavoured yoghurt with no live cultures when you can choose a creamy and nutritiously rich option packed with beneficial bacteria and add your own fresh strawberries? This is just one example that demonstrates how the way you frame your thoughts around dietary choices can make healthier options more appealing.

Dairy can be challenging for some individuals to tolerate due to the lactose content and of course if you have a dairy allergy it should be avoided completely. However, if you think you might have an intolerance and you find that too much dairy contributes to impaired bowel habits or discomfort in the gut, you might still be able to tolerate a very small amount. Incorporating even small amounts of dairy containing live cultures into the diet is ideal for topping up on key nutrients and promoting gut health. If you think you have an issue with dairy, it's always advised to seek personalised advice from a healthcare professional to assess your tolerance levels.

Herbs and Spices

The benefits of herbs and spices on our health and particularly our immune health are very much underestimated. Although often categorised together there is a distinction between herbs and spices. The leaves of the plant are referred to as the herbs and the dried elements such as the roots, seeds and bark are known as the spices.

We tend to assume that consuming herbs and spices in such minuscule amounts compared to the other foods means they can't have much of an impact on health but that is not always the case. There's a reason that for thousands of years, long before modern medicine, herbs and spices have sat within the foundation of traditional and ancient medicines and have been celebrated for their antioxidative, antimicrobial, antiviral, anti-fungal and anti-inflammatory benefits. Herbs and spices alone should not be used in place of modern medicine but, nonetheless, incorporating them into your diet regularly can assist your overall wellbeing and immune function. However, the effects of herbs and spices can be dose dependent and there are definitely risks associated with overconsumption, due to potential toxicity. Overconsumption often comes through supplements, and not what is consumed in the diet. Rather than stocking up your cupboard with capsules of ginger, garlic, turmeric and the like, focus on incorporating fresh and dried forms into your foods and expanding your palate in the process. Collectively herbs and spices appear to have beneficial health effects, but how do they marry up individually?

Turmeric

Turmeric has been used for decades to support the immune system, with some people even claiming it has anti-cancer properties. However, this claim is unproven and in many ways is an irresponsible message, since cancer is incredibly complicated and the causes are multifactorial. Yet there is some evidence to suggest that turmeric can help to promote immune health. The active ingredient in turmeric is curcumin and it's this component of the spice which is predominantly responsible for the beneficial effects of turmeric. Evidence suggests curcumin may help to reduce pain caused as a result of rheumatoid arthritis and psoriasis. Curcumin also promotes antioxidant activity, and it's thought that it may also help with managing blood sugar control. However, the dose of turmeric will affect its potential and as mentioned above high doses can contribute to adverse side effects. High doses in supplement form can also interact with a wide range of medications. So focus on adding turmeric to your vegetables, soups and curries rather than supplementing in high doses. Furthermore, the bioavailability of curcumin is low, but adding black pepper increases the amount you can absorb and utilise due to its active ingredient piperine.

Ginger

Ginger is another spice that has long been used to help ward off colds and flu and to reduce the symptoms of inflammatory-related conditions. Thankfully, there is some research to show that ginger can help to promote anti-inflammatory and antioxidative effects too. Ginger contains a variety of bioactive compounds which can impact the immune system in numerous different ways. The active component of ginger is gingerol. This is a type of polyphenol that has been identified as being partly responsible for its antioxidative effects. Ginger has also been shown to reduce the effects of reactive oxygen species (molecules which can contribute to oxidation and cell damage in the body) and oxidative stress. It also promotes analgesic effects which can help to combat nausea. Nausea is often as a result of medications, pregnancy symptoms or intense pain as a result of chronic inflammatory conditions. When you can, try to incorporate fresh ginger, ground ginger or ginger tea into your diet to support your immunity. It can also be juiced and added to sparkling water as a delicious refreshing drink.

Garlic

Along with its prebiotic properties, garlic can also support immune cell function as a result of its ability to modify the immune system. The bioactive compounds in garlic have been shown to produce beneficial antioxidative and antimicrobial effects alongside modifications to the production of cytokines. Crushed garlic has been shown to provide more bioactive compounds than whole garlic cloves so chopping or crushing your garlic into pasta sauces, curries, pies and salad dressings is a great way to increase its benefits.

Cinnamon

Cinnamon is predominantly derived from cinnamon bark and cinnamon leaves. Not only does it contain a range of bioactive compounds, it's also rich in key micronutrients such as iron, manganese and fibre and provides a naturally sweet essence to many dishes. Cinnamon has also been found to have beneficial effects on blood glucose regulation and can be a useful addition to the diet for those who are at risk of diabetes. Cinnamaldehyde, which is one of the biologically active compounds present in cinnamon, may also help reduce the effects of unwanted fungus in the gut as well as promoting anti-inflammatory effects in the gut and consequently supporting an optimal gut lining. Cinnamon can be added to a spectrum of dishes and is particularly delicious in baked goods, sprinkled onto yoghurt and porridge and used as a tea. As with all herbs and spices, cinnamon should be consumed in moderation.

Lemon and honey

I'm sure many of us have been partial to a hot lemon and honey drink as a remedy for reducing the symptoms of a common cold or flu. This is a concoction that has been passed down through generations, but is there any evidence in support of the claims? Lemons are a source of vitamin C, which does play an important role in reducing the severity of the common cold and flu. However, the concentrations in which you're consuming it in this form are unlikely to be curing your symptoms. Additionally, as the lemon is being added to hot water the heat can contribute to destroying the beneficial properties of the vitamin C. Honey does contain a variety of antioxidants and polyphenols, which can help to reduce inflammation and oxidative stress and support immune health. However, as honey is often mass-produced and imported from a variety of countries with fairly loose regulations, the quality of the honey and any potential beneficial compounds found in some of the honey on our supermarket shelves are questionable to say the least. Where possible try to ensure you're buying raw and local or organic honey since this is more likely to be of high quality and richer in biologically active compounds. That said, do be mindful that incorporating honey into the diet contributes towards the recommended maximum intake of 30g of sugar per day. Despite honey having beneficial effects on our immune system and general health it is also a high-sugar ingredient that can drive blood glucose spikes and crashes in much the same way as refined sugars.

Evidently, herbs and spices can be a very powerful and nutrient-dense addition to our diets. Alongside their micro-nutrient profiles they also contain bioactive compounds which can help to support anti-inflammatory processes within the immune system and provide nourishment for our gut microbes. Furthermore, the use of herbs and spices in cooking can provide an abundance of flavour, which consequently can reduce the need for adding excess salt to your meals. What's more, a hefty sprinkling of fresh herbs can also make a dish look very attractive.

Incorporating more herbs and spices into the diet can look like the following:

- Using fresh or dried herbs to make curries or as the base for pasta sauces.
- Adding fresh ginger or turmeric to your smoothies.
- Incorporating fresh garlic into homemade dressings and sauces.

- Adding fresh herbs such as coriander to hummus.
- Infusing fresh mint or rosemary in your water bottle.
- Adding paprika, cumin and coriander to roasted vegetables.
- Using a range of dried herbs in soups (this can also reduce the amount of stock required).
- Brewing fresh ginger, mint or turmeric in hot water for tea.

Supporting Your Immune System On the Go

The reality is that many of us are spending our days rushing from place to place, from meeting to meeting and attempting to fit in a thousand tasks at once. Unfortunately, this lifestyle can have compromising effects on all areas of our social, physical and mental wellbeing. Eating on the go is a common practice in our society and it's completely unrealistic to suggest that we all have time to sit down on a daily basis and cook each meal from scratch. So rather than intensifying the pressure to do better we need to focus on working within our means and with the resources we have available. We know that the availability of ultra-processed foods, the environment and lifestyles are playing a considerable role in our health outcomes. The irony is that although we have more information, access to education and resources to be able to make the necessary changes than any generation before us, we're the ones living in an obesogenic and unhealthy environment.

I'm here to show you that with the right tools it is possible to make small tweaks to help encourage you to consume healthier foods and optimise your lifestyle. Over the next few pages you'll find tips for how to support your immune system by incorporating some of the foods highlighted above into your busy lifestyle.

Cook once, eat twice (minimum)

My number one rule is to maximise your time and effort in the kitchen. Cooking double or triple servings at any given time can help to save your time, your money and your health. For example, if you're cooking up some brown rice, try to cook extra for lunch the next day. You can then use it to add as a base for salad, to serve with leftover curries or stews or to add to soups (which you can buy ready-made or make at home). Additionally, if you're slicing up vegetables always try to slice up more than you need so you shorten the time you spend cooking your next meal. Most vegetables can be frozen raw and then used for adding to soups, stews, curries or roasting.

Take advantage of healthier on-the-go options

Picking up food on the go doesn't necessarily mean grabbing a fast-food takeaway. Most supermarkets have ready-to-go food options which can include sandwiches made with wholegrain bread (be mindful of the fillings), salads (although be conscious of your dressings), pre-chopped vegetables which you can enjoy with a small tub of hummus or salsa and fruit. When you're look-ing at sandwiches, try to opt for one with a good-quality protein source that is low in saturated fats, for example, salmon, tuna, chicken, egg or chickpeas. Additionally, do be aware of the salt and sugar content of any added sauces, chutneys or mayonnaise.

If you're buying a prepared salad, try to choose one with a dressing on the side as dressings can be high in salt and sugar; this way you can moderate how much you're adding. Alternatively, if you're eating at your desk, you can add your own vinegar or olive oil. You can also always opt for pre-cooked chicken or fish or the tinned varieties to top up on your protein and healthy fats.

Be mindful of your snacks

Despite the fact that the food industry is constantly pushing us towards snacking, it's a habit that many people are striving to break. Snacking itself isn't necessarily an undesirable habit; in fact, it can be a really useful break in the day to provide extra fuel that'll see you through the rest of the morning or afternoon, and the perfect opportunity to top up on your micronutrients and nourish your gut with some extra plants. Therefore, more influential to our health than the habit itself, is what we're snacking on and how we're snacking. Snacking on high-sugar foods throughout the day contributes to blood glucose spikes and crashes, which not only impacts your concentration, energy and mood but, over a prolonged period of time, can also contribute to low level chronic inflammation. Snacking, however, can be the perfect opportunity to top up on your micronutrients and nourish your gut with some extra plants.

Snacking is very different to grazing. A snack should be a designated stop in the day to take a break, sit down and enjoy an item of food which feels substantial and satiating. Grazing, however, is a behaviour which involves the constant eating of small amounts of food throughout the day. Often there is no designated time for grazing and it occurs too regularly throughout the day. Consistent grazing habits can drive a blood glucose rollercoaster and the secretion of insulin. Grazing can also lead to overeating, as continually picking at small amounts of food can equate to a substantial intake throughout the day. Additionally, you're more likely to graze mindlessly too and, consequently, you're unlikely to feel as full as you would if you were to sit down with a more significant snack.

If you are someone who enjoys a snack mid-morning or in the afternoons, do try to approach this in the same manner as you would a meal. Take a break from your tasks and spend five or ten minutes with your snack, enjoying it and savouring it before heading back to your daily tasks. As we discussed in Chapter 3, mindful eating can allow you to feel more satiated and fuller for longer. It can also help to support digestion and promotes nutrient absorption, which is vital for optimising your immunity.

Alternatively, some individuals prefer to eat three main meals per day. If you're someone who isn't much of a snacker, that's no bad thing. This section isn't about encouraging you to snack if you don't feel the need or desire to. But if you are struggling with low energy levels or are feeling slightly depleted throughout the day then it may be something you want to consider introducing slowly.

Opting for a healthy snack can definitely be more challenging at times, since our environment is constantly encouraging us to opt for those less nutritious options. For example, lunchtime meal deals in supermarkets are a common marketing strategy. Since the meal deal price of the main, drink and snack is significantly less than buying these items individually, it's often the lower value snacks, which tend to be higher in sugar and saturated fats, that are included. Unfortunately, the same goes for the drinks and, as a result, it can be really tempting to pick up a chocolate bar, bag of crisps or a cookie and a high-sugar or artificially sweetened fizzy drink with lunch, particularly when it makes your overall lunch more cost-effective. However, you're better off opting for a bottle of water if a meal deal is the most cost-effective way to buy lunch.

The good news is that there are alternative options to high-sugar snacks. Many supermarkets do include some nutritious snacks in their meal deals, though admittedly the choice is often more limited. These often include hard-boiled eggs, sliced fruit and carrot sticks and hummus.

You could also try packing a snack for work or when you're out and about. There are some delicious and nutritious snack recipes at the back of the book (see page 245) for you to take with you on the go.

Moreover, if you're spending time at home, your snacks can become more adventurous. Here are a few quick and easy immune-supporting snacks for you to try.

- Smashed avocado on oatcakes.
- Cream cheese or hummus on rice cakes.
- Greek yoghurt with berries and cinnamon.
- Sliced banana with peanut, cashew or almond butter.
- Roasted chickpeas.

Should we be buying organic produce?

There's been a growing interest in organic food, due in part to concern about the use of fertilisers and pesticides in modern-day farming methods. Consequently, these considerations are driving a greater focus on the beneficial effects of consuming a diet based around organic foods.

Although the regulations on organic produce do vary by country, the general premise of organic farming is that no artificial pesticides or synthetic fertilisers are used to grow the produce.

Surprisingly, the evidence on the benefits of organic is relatively limited. However, what we do have suggests that the nutritional values of organic crops are higher than those produced through non-organic farming methods. The evidence points to increased levels of phytonutrients and vitamins and minerals in the organic varieties. However, when it comes to nutrition and diet, nutritional quality isn't the only consideration when making dietary choices.

Post-pandemic the cost of living is rising drastically and consuming a healthy balanced diet based on whole foods is becoming more and more expensive. The promotion of organic produce adds to the notion that consuming a healthy diet to support immune health and general wellbeing is elitist. Yet eating nourishing foods to support your long-term immune function, physical and mental health does not have to be cripplingly expensive. The message to you is to work within your means, rather than aiming for standards which are unachievable.

It's easy to get caught up in the less important areas of your diet at the expense of avoiding overconsuming high-sugar, higher-fat foods. By this I mean it's not uncommon to fixate on the microdetails of consuming organic vs non-organic or sourcing the finest kefir, when the basics of your diet could still do with a significant amount of work.

However, if the idea of organic produce appeals to you and you can afford some – but not all – organic produce,

where possible opt for those fruits and vegetables that
don't have a protective skin, e.g. berries, apples, nectarines,
spinach, peppers and tomatoes. If your budget allows,
switching to organic or ethically produced eggs, meat, fish
and dairy will also be beneficial.

The Role of Seasonal Eating in Immune Health

Eating seasonally is the concept of eating certain produce at the
time of its peak harvest. Seasonal eating is something which is
often associated with those who are more in touch with nature,
their health and the environment, but it's something which
many of us should be making a conscious effort to incorporate into our diets and lifestyles. Alongside the role that eating
seasonally can have on supporting our immunity and general
physiological function (which I'll come to), it can have many
other benefits too.

Seasonal produce is typically higher in micronutrients, antioxidants and phytochemicals as the soil quality and nutritional
status varies at different times of the year in order to produce
various fruits and vegetables. Since such produce typically
doesn't spend a prolonged period of time travelling across con-
tinents there's less time for the degradation of nutrients and
phytochemicals. Eating seasonally also means we're more likely
to consume the produce closer to its harvest date than when it's
transported halfway across the world.

Furthermore, consuming certain fruits and vegetables at
specific times of the year is a great way to meet our nutritional
requirements, which can vary throughout the months. For

example, citrus fruits such as oranges are in peak season during the winter months and are a rich source of vitamin C, which is required to help reduce the severity and duration of illnesses such as the common cold and flu. Winter is the prime time for starchy vegetables such as parsnips, sweet potatoes, butternut squash and potatoes. This makes perfect sense for satisfying our need for more starchy, comforting and hearty foods during these months. Additionally, higher water content produce tends to be in season throughout the summer months. This is particularly beneficial in supporting our hydration requirements during the summer as we lose more fluid due to increased sweating. It's also no coincidence that lettuce, courgettes, cucumbers and tomatoes tend to be at their peak during the summer months, as we tend to desire lighter and more refreshing meals.

Consuming produce out of season means it's less likely to contain the quantities of the nutrients we require at that time of year. This is because produce consumed out of season is often encouraged to ripen unnaturally and therefore may skip the vital aspects of nutrient development. In contrast, seasonal produce tends to have more flavour due to being able to ripen at its most natural time. As a result tomatoes will be juicer in the summer and autumn months and strawberries will be naturally sweeter during the summer period.

Another important benefit of eating seasonally is that it can encourage us to try new produce and incorporate a wider variety of foods into the diet. This in turn can support our nutritional requirements as well as providing a greater degree of diversity for the gut and immune system.

While eating seasonally has clear benefits for our immune system, it's also a more environmentally friendly way of eating, not only because of the reduction in transportation but also because the produce requires less refrigeration. Both of these factors play their part in the overall cost, therefore sourcing food more locally can make it more affordable. As a result, eating seasonally can not only help to protect your pocket but can help to support the local farmers and communities in the process.

Finally, eating seasonally doesn't have to be a full commitment. Simply becoming a little more aware of the sources of your food and dipping in and out of eating seasonally can help to reduce unnecessary transportation and provide you with an even more nutritious diet.

There's a lot of information in this chapter and if you're not familiar with some of it, it may seem a little overwhelming. However, incorporating these foods into your diet doesn't necessarily mean you need to overhaul everything all at once. It's always more effective in the long run to gradually add more whole foods into your diet as these can naturally displace some of those higher-sugar, more processed varieties. This way you're more likely to be able to make sustainable changes for the long term. You may choose to take one or two tips included in this chapter and introduce them into your diet each week. For example, next time you're making a Bolognese simply try adding a tin of lentils or beans to the sauce.

As we've discussed above, thinking about your snacking habits can also be a really simple but effective way to incorporate more of these whole foods into your diet. Simple changes such as being prepared with a snack for work or adding a tub of hummus and some oatcakes to your shopping list can bring your intentions to life.

It's also important to re-highlight that food should first and foremost be something that you enjoy, so this isn't about encouraging you to eat foods you don't like. It's about encouraging you to explore new foods and incorporate them into your diet in different ways. The truth is, very few people enjoy a side of boiled cauliflower but try roasting it in the oven and drizzling over a tahini dressing with some fresh mint and pomegranate seeds and you've got a completely different taste experience (and a whole lot more nutrients too!).

Summary Points

- Fruits such as apples, pears and peaches are rich in pectin, a type of fibre which has been associated with immune-mediating effects on the production of cytokines. Pectin can also help to support the growth of the good bacteria in the gut.
- Incorporating more wholegrains into the diet can help you to hit the recommended intake of 30g of fibre per day. The consumption of wholegrains has been associated with a range of beneficial health outcomes.
- Oily fish and some nuts, such as walnuts, can contribute to an increase in omega-3 intake.
- Adding more herbs and spices to your diet can help to reduce your salt intake and increase your consumption of plant compounds. Consuming a diverse range of herbs and spices contributes significantly to supporting variety in the diet.
- Eggs contain key nutrients such as choline, vitamin D, proteins, selenium and zinc. These nutrients are required to support immune cell function.

- Snacking mindfully can be a useful way to support your nutritional requirements and immune system. Try to avoid high-sugar snacks and opt for those high in protein and fibre instead.
- Eating seasonally can help to provide the immune system with the relevant nutrients required at specific times of the year.

CHAPTER 7

Dietary Components Hindering Our Immunity

In the previous chapter we looked at foods which we should focus on increasing in the diet. This chapter is all about those common dietary components that can hinder our immunity. These are the foods that we want to try to limit in the diet. Limiting certain foods is best done by displacing them with more nutritious options.

This brings us back to a primary ethos of this book: striking a balance between your physical, mental and social wellbeing. It's important to note that some foods which can negatively affect your immune function and physical health may be the same foods that can contribute to supporting your social wellbeing. So how can we create a balance between supporting our physical wellbeing while also nourishing our desires? Focusing on limiting certain foods rather than removing them entirely can help to guide us towards a better balance. Removing complete food groups can pose risks of nutritional deficiencies and may contribute to feelings of restriction, isolation and poorer mental wellbeing. In contrast, limiting these foods can help to reduce their negative effects on the immune system and general phys-ical health while still positively contributing to supporting our mental and social wellbeing every now and again.

Which Foods Should We Try to Limit?

Sugar

It's no surprise that sugar is top of the list here. Sugar is vastly overconsumed in our modern diets as it's managed to find its way into the majority of food products on our supermarket shelves. In the UK the recommended maximum intake is 30g per day, which is equivalent to around 6 teaspoons, but the latest find-ings from the UK's National Diet and Nutrition Survey suggests that female adults are consuming an average of 44g per day and males an average of 55.5g per day.

It's tricky to avoid sugar as it is no longer an ingredient confined to sweet snacks, desserts and ice cream. It's branched out into products which are perceived as healthy too, so these days it's likely that everything from your bread, cereals, cereal bars, yoghurts, pasta sauces to ready meals, savoury snacks and flavoured waters, and numerous products in between, contain sugar. As a result, it's extremely challenging to move away from and even limit our sugar intakes. Often the best place to start is by capping those typically sweet foods – think cake, sweets and chocolate – as limiting it elsewhere is far more challenging when you're trying to consume a normal diet that includes convenient items such as ready-made pasta sauces, breakfast cereals and toast, many of which contain sugar.

Sugar isn't entirely harmful as we do need small amounts of it to support our glucose requirements. However, this sugar is best sourced from natural sources such as complex carbohydrates. In terms of immune function, the immune cells require glucose to provide the energy that allows them to function optimally. For example, when the immune system is activated in response to a threat, chemokines (proteins which send signals around the body) send chemical messages to the macrophages (white blood cells) to signal for help. The macrophages then trigger the response of the T-cells and B-cells for them to attend the site of attack. In order for this cascade of responses to occur, adequate glucose stores are essential.

Yet, finding that sweet spot for your glucose reserves is vital, as overly elevated levels in the blood can cause adverse effects to the immune system. Short-term hyperglycaemia (high levels of sugar in the blood) can alter the way in which the immune cells respond to an intruder and consequently may adversely affect the outcome of an infection. These hindrances include a reduced ability for the white blood cells to move around, impairments in the abilities of white blood cells to destroy unwanted pathogens and delayed messenger responses. Put together, you can see how these effects can impair the immune response and its ability to fight intruders.

If the hyperglycaemia is prolonged, long-term changes to the adaptive immune cells can occur. This can negatively alter the way in which the adaptive immune cells respond altogether.

Animal studies have shown that long-term hyperglycaemia can cause glycation and glycoxidation to the proteins within the immune system. Glycation is a process whereby sugars bind to the protein, which prevents their normal function, while glycoxidation is the oxidation of the sugars, which can also have destructive effects on the immune cells. The dendritic cells, which are partly responsible for capturing unwanted pathogens, are also hindered by the effects of hyperglycaemia. Mice studies have shown that impaired dendritic cells can attack the usually friendly apo-B protein (a component of low-density lipoprotein cholesterol and triglycerides). Over time, this may contribute to an increased risk of autoimmune type responses.

Furthermore, prolonged hyperglycaemia can cause an increased inflammatory response and damage to the beta-cells. Beta-cells are responsible for the production of insulin and when they become damaged there can be an increased risk of type 2 diabetes and low-grade chronic inflammation.

However, the picture isn't all that simple. On the flipside, when glucose levels are too low there's an increased risk of hypo-glycaemia (low levels of sugar in the blood) and in such cases the activities of the immune cells are suppressed too. Consequently, both too high or too low blood sugar levels can be detrimental in supporting immune function.

Controlling blood glucose levels is undeniably essential in supporting immune cell function. A vast array of evidence has highlighted the implications of impaired blood glucose control on immune function and the risk of disease in both healthy and critically ill individuals. Ultimately, it's all about finding the right balance.

We've seen the direct impacts sugar can have on the immune system and some research suggests that an overconsumption of sugar may also contribute to alterations in the gut microbes. Discovering the full extent of these alterations requires far more research. We do know that the relationship between the gut microbiome and sugar intake can be a bidirectional one. Not only can sugar impact the types of microbes present in the gut, the gut can also influence the desire for high-sugar foods.

Identifying sugar in your food products is a challenge in itself since there are hundreds of different sources and names for sugar. The list below includes just some of the many examples, but familiarising yourself with this non-exhaustive list can help you to spot many of the more common ones.

beet syrup	fruit juice concentrate	maple syrup	glucose syrup
agave syrup	corn syrup	date syrup	rice syrup
invert syrup	simple syrup	molasses	high-fructose corn syrup
honey	cane juice	cane sugar	unrefined cane sugar
sucrose	fructose	dextrose	maltose

Some foods contain natural sugars from whole fruits or vegetables. Therefore reading the ingredients list alongside the nutrition tables on food packs can help you to identify whether the sugars are added or come from more natural sources. Additionally, the values in the 'of which sugars' section of the nutritional values table can provide a further insight. Products containing less than 5g of sugar per 100g are classified as low-sugar products, while those containing more than 22.5g per 100g are considered high-sugar products. It's the higher and moderate sugar products which we should be limiting in our diet.

Limiting sugar in your diet is far more achievable than is often believed. Many of us have conditioned ourselves to believe that we require a sweet snack at specific times of the day to see us through. But the more sugar we eat, the more we'll crave as our taste buds can become less sensitive to sweet foods. Rather than going cold turkey, it's best to cut back slowly as this can help to recondition the taste buds so that your food doesn't taste quite so bland. Below are a few tips on how you can moderate your sugar intake:

- Halve the amount of sugar in your tea and coffee.
- Switch your afternoon biscuits to a handful of nuts, natural yoghurt with fresh berries or crackers with hummus.
- Switch your high-sugar cereals to homemade granola or a lower sugar option.
- Avoid fat-free products as these are often high in sugar or artificial sweeteners.
- Opt for natural yoghurt over flavoured yoghurt and season with cinnamon.
- Check the ingredients of your sauces for hidden sugars; where possible, try to make them at home.
- Switch fruit juices for water, fruit-infused water or herbal teas.

Furthermore, by naturally reducing high-sugar foods in your diet you're making more space for those highly nutritious whole foods that we are aiming to increase. Replacing foods with a more nutritious alternative can be a much more positive way of looking at your diet, rather than thinking about removing foods in isolation.

Controlling blood glucose levels

In addition to reducing overall sugar intake, controlling blood glucose levels is also pivotal to supporting immune function. Your blood glucose response can be massively impacted by certain food combinations and the order in which you eat your food. Here are some tips which can help you optimise blood glucose control:

- **Combine your carbohydrates with a source of protein**
  Adding a source of protein to your carbohydrate sources can help to slow down the release of sugar into the bloodstream and minimise spikes in blood glucose concentrations. For example, when snacking, try consuming a spoonful of peanut butter along with an apple, a handful of nuts with your dried fruit or a few squares of chocolate. When thinking about lunch or dinner, you could try adding tuna to a jacket potato, seeds or a tahini dressing to roasted root vegetables or flaked salmon to pasta dishes. Adding egg whites, nut butter, Greek yoghurt or mixed seeds to a bowl of porridge at breakfast can support blood glucose regulation and satiety too.

- **Eat your greens first**
  The order in which you eat the food on your plate can have an impact on blood glucose levels. Always go for the green vegetables first, followed by the protein source, healthy fats and then the simple or complex carbohydrates. The fibre in the vegetables, protein and healthy fats will slow down the rate of the release of sugars from the carbohydrates.

- **Engage in movement after eating**
  Walking after a meal can help to lower blood glucose levels as the activation of the muscles utilises some of the glucose in the blood, which consequently causes blood sugar to fall. Try to go for a 10–15-minute walk after lunch and dinner (this becomes far easier in the summer months where the evenings are warmer and lighter).

- **Consuming vinegar ahead of a meal**
  Evidence suggests that diluting vinegar in water before a carbohydrate-rich meal can lower the impact of the

carbohydrates on blood glucose. The acetic acid in the vinegar increases the utilisation of glucose by the muscles and consequently lowers the concentration of glucose in the blood. The recommended dose is 1–2 tablespoons diluted in water, and it's recommended to drink this through a straw to protect your teeth from the effects of the acid. While this may help with blood glucose regulation, it's not always feasible or socially acceptable if we're eating out or on the go, so don't feel it should become a non-negotiable behaviour before every meal. Consequently, this may be more relevant to those who struggle with blood glucose control.

- **Be aware of the effects of 'healthy foods' on blood glucose control**

  Foods that are often seen as 'healthy', such as sweetened oat milks, juices and flavoured yoghurts, can often creep into our daily diets. These foods also include cereals often perceived as healthy (e.g. some granolas and similar options containing added syrups), but they're notorious for their impact on spiking blood glucose. Where possible, if you're using dairy-free milks, opt for unsweetened soya milk or nut milk as an alternative to oat milk, which can be higher in sugar. Pick smoothies over juices and ensure your cereals are made with wholegrains, as these are higher in fibre than refined alternatives.

Being aware of these behaviours and habits can help to encourage slight changes in the way in which you're eating and consequently can elicit a more positive effect on blood glucose regulation.

None of this advice means you have to decline the cake and

catch-up with a friend or relative or completely drop the pick and mix at the cinema. It's more about looking at your diet as a whole and trying to focus on eating whole foods 80–90 per cent of the time and then enjoying those higher-sugar foods every now and again ... just not every day.

Can artificial sweeteners be used as a healthier alternative?

In Chapter 3 we touched on the impact of artificial sweeteners on our gut microbes. Here we're taking a deeper dive to assess how artificial sweeteners may influence the physiological function of the immune cells.

As we try to move towards a lower-sugar diet, we're often searching for alternatives for our favourite products; many or most of these will use artificial sweeteners to create the sweet taste we're so accustomed to. These alternatives are often the products labelled 'sugar-free' and include things like sugar-free squash, sugar-free yoghurt, sugar-free sweets and so on. The most common artificial sweeteners found in our food products include aspartame, acesulfame K, saccharin and sucralose, to name just a few.

Artificial sweeteners are also referred to as non-nutritive sweeteners as they lack nutritional value and calories, while at the same time being anywhere between 200 and 20,000 times sweeter than white sugar. Since artificial sweeteners have no calorific value, ironically they're often associated with perceived healthier eating patterns and consequently some evidence has found that those who consume a diet in line with the healthy eating guidelines are also more likely to be consuming artificial sweeteners. However, this may be down to misleading marketing messages surrounding artificial sweeteners.

Artificial sweeteners enable products to maintain their sweet taste while simultaneously keeping energy levels low. This provides marketers with an even stronger messaging strategy as it allows them to claim these products are lower in calories. From an industry perspective this sounds like a total win. So much so that it sounds too good to be true (it is!). Here I'll explain how, in some cases, the mass food industries' priorities and our individual health requirements aren't always aligned. Perhaps artificial sweeteners may not be as sweet as they taste after all.

Recent research on mice has shown that high intakes of sucralose can affect the membrane signalling of T-cells and may limit T-cell proliferation and differentiation. This means that the ability of T-cells to increase in number and their ability to differentiate into a variety of roles is impaired. Furthermore, the research showed a reduced efficiency of T-cell receptors, which can negatively impact the adaptive immune system. Additionally, the overconsumption of artificial sweeteners can cause increases in the secretion of inflammatory cytokines. Although the dose and type of sweetener can influence how the immune cells respond to artificial sweeteners, the research certainly does indicate negative effects of artificial sweeteners on immunity.

Furthermore, as we explored in Chapter 3, animal studies have shown that some artificial sweeteners can contribute to changes to the gut microbiome and may also contribute to dysbiosis and increased inflammation in the gut and the gut lining, all of which can have indirect implications in altering the immune response. Some research has shown that the changes caused to the gut microbes in response to overconsuming artificial sweeteners may also affect blood glucose control. While they may not appear to directly influence our blood sugar levels at the time of consumption, if artificial sweeteners are overconsumed in the long term, they can have detrimental effects on overall blood glucose control.

In response to the latest developments in the research, in May 2023 the World Health Organization released new guidelines suggesting that artificial sweeteners should not be used as a mechanism for weight management or to reduce the risk of non-communicable diseases.

The degree to which artificial sweeteners are present in so many products and the quantities in which we're consuming them may have negative implications on our gut health and our immune response. As a result, it's important to try to limit artificial sweeteners where you can. You can do this by implementing the following changes:

- Avoid adding artificial sweeteners to your tea and coffee.
- Limit the consumption of 'sugar-free' sweets and chewing gum.
- Limit the consumption of foods marketed as 'fat-free', as many of these are likely to contain artificial sweeteners.
- Switch diet versions of fizzy drinks for kombucha or sparkling water.

It's worth noting that while we continue to replace sugar in our diets with artificial sweeteners, our taste receptors will still be seeking out that sweet hit and thus the desire for sweet foods is unlikely to subside. Unfortunately, artificial sweeteners are commonly found in processed and ultra-processed foods and so for as long as we use artificial sweeteners in this way we'll continue to feel the need for highly processed and ultra-processed foods.

Food additives

Food additives are substances which are added to food for a functional benefit. These benefits can include extending the shelf life, improving the palatability, texture or taste of a product, altering the appearance or colour or providing bulk to a food item.

In some cases, food additives are used for nutritionally beneficial purposes such as fortification; the most common examples include ascorbic acid (vitamin C), folic acid (vitamin B9) or vitamin D. However, in the majority of cases food additives are used for reasons other than to improve the nutritional quality of the product. In such cases these ingredients may have more harmful effects on our health than first meets the eye.

All food additives undergo rigorous testing for safety and adverse health implications, in which the results determine their safety of use and upper limits permitted for use in food products. However, due to the industrialisation of our food industry, these additives are creeping into far more of our products than we generally realise. As with artificial sweeteners, which are also considered as food additives, the routine consumption of food additives in small amounts can contribute to adverse effects on our health and immune system. Furthermore, animal studies have shown that food additives can play havoc with the ability to metabolise food effectively and manage blood glucose control. Of course, specific food additives will have varying effects on our health. Let's look at the impact of some of the common food additives on our health and immune system:

- **Titanium dioxide** This food additive has no nutritional value, it simply provides the white colour to products such as icing, toothpaste, sweets and chewing gum and is also known as E171. (Funny how food additives don't sound as intimidating or catastrophic when there's a number attached to them rather than a harsh sounding chemical.) It was deemed safe in the EU and Northern Ireland by the Food Standards Agency until February 2022; however, there were concerns about the long-term implications of the nano-sized particles and the potential of bioaccumulation when consumed on a regular basis, despite the relatively low individual doses. Furthermore, it's believed that the minuscule particle sizes of titanium dioxide can contribute to impaired absorption in the gut and mice studies have shown that regular intake, even at a low dose, can disrupt immune function through increasing inflammation and the production of reactive oxygen species. It's also thought that titanium dioxide may assist in DNA damage. Although it's no longer used in the EU and Northern Ireland, it is still legal in other countries around the world so it's always worth reading labels if you travel regularly.

- **Carrageenan** This food additive is used for its thickening and stabilising properties and can be identified on food labels as E407. The chronic exposure of carrageenan has been shown to negatively affect metabolic homeostasis (i.e. maintaining the normal balance of metabolism) and the permeability of the gut lining. Carrageenan is also commonly utilised alongside emulsifiers, which can aid its absorption; this combination becomes a recipe for additional adverse effects on the permeability of the gut lining. Since carrageenan is often present in ultra-processed, high-fat foods such as whipped cream, ultra-processed desserts and chocolate yoghurts, the combination of the saturated fats and the carrageenan can further influence the permeability of the gut lining.

- **Allura Red** Otherwise known as E129, Allura Red provides the red colouring in many sweets, cakes and soft drinks. It is well understood for its role in contributing to hyperactivity in children, particularly in those with ADHD, and more recent research has shown that a high consumption of E129 can increase the risk of inflammatory bowel disease and allergies in children. Limiting the consumption of E129 may help to modify the effects on behaviour and reduce the risks of adverse effects on immune function.

- **Monosodium glutamate (MSG)** MSG, otherwise known as E621, is an incredibly overutilised food additive that is exploited for its flavour-enhancing properties. MSG is found so widely in the products on our supermarket shelves that there are significant concerns surrounding its overconsumption. MSG is often found in foods high in saturated fats and trans fats. The combination of fats with MSG contributes to metabolic dysregulation, systemic abnormalities and impaired activity of the immune system. An overconsumption has also been associated with an increased production in reactive oxygen species and an inflammatory response. The production of the reactive oxygen species can alter redox homeostasis, a process which is essential for regulating the complexities of everyday physiological functioning and protecting against the adverse effects of reactive oxygen species. Redox homeostasis is vital in regulating the function of the immune system. Furthermore, MSG has the power to alter appetite hormones and can drive an increased desire for high-fat foods. Over a prolonged period of time this can contribute to an increase in the risk of obesity.

- **Emulsifiers** These are used for a variety of purposes such as combining substances which would usually separate from each other (such as oil from water), slowing the melting rate of ice cream and increasing texture in dough. Two common emulsifiers include carboxymethylcellulose (CMC), which is also known as cellulose gum, and polysorbate-80 (P-80). P-80 is commonly found in food ingredients lists as E433. Both CMC and P-80 are approved food additives and are considered safe in very low concentrations. Mice studies have shown that regular low intakes were associated with low-grade inflammation, an increased risk of obesity and metabolic dysregulation. Furthermore, emulsifiers can have a potential adverse effect on dysbiosis in the gut microbiome, which can increase the potential for intestinal inflammation. The cascade in response to emulsifier-induced dysbiosis has been shown to reduce the production of short-chain fatty acids (specifically butyrate). Additionally, mice studies have also found that emulsifiers can stimulate appetite, which in turn can contribute to a further risk of obesity. It's unknown whether the emulsifiers themselves have a direct effect on appetite regulatory hormones or whether the changes in the gut microbiome modify the regulation of appetite hormones.

It's worth noting that the majority of the research around the health implications of food additives are conducted on rodents due to the ethical complexities of conducting these studies on humans (of course we'll all have our own opinions on the ethics associated with animal studies too). Consequently, it's challenging to directly imply the same to be true for humans and we do need more evidence. However, the research we have suggests that food additives can have adverse effects on our gut health, inflammatory markers and our immune cell function. Similarly to sugar, eliminating food additives entirely can be challenging as many of them are used for functional purposes. However, by largely focusing on a diet based around whole foods you'll naturally notice a reduction in the consumption of food additives. Foods we consume outside of the home and in restaurants are more likely to contain these ingredients yet we still want to enjoy eating out, therefore try to limit foods containing these ingredients at home to reduce your total intakes.

Salt

It's no surprise that as salt is one of the most prevalent ingredients in our food products today, many of us are drastically overconsuming it. For years the public health message has been that we should all be focusing on reducing our salt intake. The latest findings from the UK's 2019 National Diet and Nutrition Survey demonstrate that both male and female adults are consuming more than the recommended maximum intake of 6g per day. On average, men and women are consuming on average around 8.3g and 6.8g a day respectively.

Getting our salt intake in the right ballpark is vital as too much is detrimental, while a small amount does actually play an important role in maintaining normal physiological function. For this reason, trying to remove salt from the diet completely can be equally as problematic as eating too much of it.

Salt consists of sodium and chloride, two key electrolytes which have very functional roles in the body. Sodium plays an important role in maintaining fluid balance and hydration, as well as supporting muscle function and the nervous system.

Salt deficiency can lead to an increased risk of hyponatraemia, which can occur when the body does not have enough sodium. The consequential effects can include headaches, nausea, vomiting, lack of energy and fatigue, muscle cramps and – in severe cases – seizures and coma. Conversely, chronically high intakes of salt can contribute to a significant increased risk of high blood pressure and cardiovascular disease. In the short term, one may also experience increased thirst and water retention following high salt intake.

In relation to the immune system, a chronically high salt intake has also been shown to increase the risks of autoimmune diseases and inflammation in mice studies. Human studies have also shown an increase in monocytes and proinflammatory cytokines in response to a high salt diet. In this case the researchers were using 12g of salt per day, which is double the maximum recommended intake. However, when salt intake was reduced there was a reduction in the proinflammatory cytokines and an increase in anti-inflammatory cytokines. The research suggests that consuming a high-salt diet may disturb immune function homeostasis, while over a prolonged period of time, a high salt intake may contribute to an increased risk of inflammation.

Since the food industry overuses salt in their products, the overconsumption of salt is far more prevalent than not consuming enough. In the UK, foods containing more than 1.5g of salt per 100g are classified as a high-salt product, while those containing less than 0.3g per 100g are considered a low-salt product.

Becoming more aware of where the hidden salt is in your food is the first step to reducing salt intake. Here are some simple steps to help you moderate your intake:

- Avoid adding salt to your food at the table.
- Use more herbs and spices in your cooking.
- Limit salted snacks such as crisps and nuts and opt for unsalted versions where possible.
- Try to limit takeaways and moderate how regularly you're eating out. Processed food and food bought outside the home tends to be the source of most of our dietary salt.
- Avoid adding salt to fries.
- Be aware of what's in your sauces and condiments. Opting for lower salt options where you can will still enable you to enjoy your favourite accompaniments, but in a healthier way.
- Limit the consumption of energy drinks as these can be a source of extra sodium.
- Avoid buying products in brine.
- Be aware of foods preserved with salt. These include olives, anchovies, miso-flavoured products and cured fish and meats. This isn't to say you should never enjoy them, but being aware of their salt content in the context of the rest of your diet is key.

For the most part, it's unlikely that you're not consuming enough salt; however, if you're cooking largely from scratch and you're not using salt in your cooking then there may be a risk of low intake. Additionally, those who engage in lots of physical activity can lose excess sweat and electrolytes as a result and for this reason may require extra salt intake. For those individuals, a rehydration drink containing extra electrolytes following an extended bout of exercise is often advised; the same applies on very hot days, which may also induce more sweating. If you're concerned about under-consuming salt on these occasions you may want to add a pinch of salt to your water or meals.

Saturated fats

In Chapter 5 we discussed the important role of fats in supporting a healthy immune function but, as we've already explored, not all fats are equal. Incorporating monounsaturated and polyunsaturated fats in the diet is hugely beneficial when it comes to supporting healthy immune function but the overconsumption of saturated fats may not be quite so favourable.

Saturated fats are defined by their chemical structure: they do not contain any double hydrogen bonds. They're typically hard when they're at room temperature and are found in a variety of foods such as cakes, biscuits, butter, ghee, red and processed meats, coconut, pies, cream and cheese. Many foods contain a combination of unsaturated and saturated fats.

Adults in the UK are advised to consume no more than 10 per cent of their total energy intake from saturated fats. However, the most recent findings from the National Diet and Nutrition Survey demonstrate that as a population we are significantly exceeding these limits. Teenagers are consuming around 12.6 per cent of their total energy intake from saturated fats. Adults aged between nineteen and sixty-four are consuming 12.3 per cent with the over seventy-fives consuming the highest amounts of saturated fat, accounting for, on average, 14.1 per cent of their total energy intake.

In Chapter 3 we saw how saturated fats can impair the integrity of the gut lining, but they may be having a detrimental impact on other aspects of the immune system too. The overconsumption of saturated fats has been linked rather conclusively to a significant increase in the risk of many inflammatory diseases such as heart disease, metabolic syndrome, obesity, atherosclerosis and type 2 diabetes. In addition to the total consumption of saturated fats, the research suggests that the balance between unsaturated and saturated fat intake may also impact the ability of the immune system to work optimally. The following tips can help reduce your saturated fat intake:

- Switch processed meats for fresh meat varieties, e.g. processed burgers for homemade turkey or chicken burgers.
- Switch biscuits in the afternoon for oatcakes.
- Swap your beef mince for chicken and turkey mince.
- Avoid frying your food and switch to grilling instead.
- Be cautious of the amount of butter you're using on toast and in your cooking.
- Try to trim fat off your cuts of meat such as lamb, steak and pork.
- Try to limit ultra-processed and fried foods in the diet.

Factors That Influence Our Dietary Choices

All of the dietary components I've discussed in this chapter can contribute to hindering immunity. However, it's important to remember that there are so many more factors that can impact our dietary choices than simply knowing what is good for us. As a result, it's important we consider these in our decision-making processes too.

It's really common to believe that the answer to making healthier dietary choices lies with strong willpower. Frankly, it can feel much easier to blame willpower than to dig any deeper into the other factors that truly influence our dietary habits. Becoming aware of these influences may help us to understand them better. It's this awareness which can allow us to incorporate tools to try to better manage these external contributing factors.

Flavour, texture, appearance and smell are some of the most important factors which influence our dietary decisions. These elements are hugely valuable as they can contribute to the enjoyment and satisfaction which we get from our food. We will all have different taste preferences, which come from a collection of variables. For example, what your mother ate throughout pregnancy and the food you were exposed to as a young child, along with memories and your genetic makeup can all contribute to influencing the types of food you enjoy eating.

Convenience and cost are also considerations when making dietary decisions. Do we have the time, money, tools and ability to cook from scratch or is it more convenient to pick up a ready-made meal? Ready-made meals are not always a less nutritious option and there are some excellent products available nowadays, but they do often come at a higher price, which can feed into the notion that consuming a healthy diet is elitist. Let's not ignore the fact that consuming a healthy diet can be perceived to be more expensive. Typically, higher-energy, higher-fat convenience foods come with a lower price and may often be found as part of a 'buy one get one free' offer. There's no denying that all this can make it even more challenging to make healthier choices. Yet with time, effort, knowledge and skill it is possible to consume a healthy balanced diet on a lower budget. One of my aims with this book is to show you how you can put some of these tips into practice with little effort, on a lower budget and with restricted time.

The food and food marketing industries are some of the greatest contributing components that drive our dietary preferences. Food advertising is a major influence on our dietary choices – we're constantly exposed to food adverts via the internet, social media, TV and the radio. As a result, our ears, eyes and minds are constantly being encouraged towards making less healthy decisions. However, becoming aware of the food marketing which we're constantly exposed to can make it easier to resist, as we may be able to transfer the messaging from the subconscious to the conscious mind. As a result, questioning our dietary choices becomes more achievable.

Demographics can also influence the food we choose to eat. As we age or reach different stages in life, our dietary preferences can change. Additionally, our occupations and social norms can also contribute to driving certain dietary patterns. For example, individuals with physically demanding jobs will require more energy than those who work at a desk. Furthermore, we can't underestimate the impact of the dietary choices and attitudes towards food and health of those around us. The behaviours and opinions of our family, friends and colleagues can influence our dietary decisions in both positive and negative ways. If someone is encouraging us to make healthier choices and leading by example, making those decisions can feel less isolating and far more manageable. In contrast, if we're close to someone who constantly tries to encourage poor dietary behaviours it can become more challenging to stick to those healthier choices. Unfortunately, the lack of support or encouragement from others to eat less nutritious foods can be a way in which other people make themselves feel better about their own dietary decisions and behaviours.

Religion and culture are other major factors which influence dietary choices and dietary patterns and this will have more of an impact for some people than others. Traditional dishes, foods and religious gatherings can drastically sway dietary choices. In some cases, certain foods may be encouraged whereas in others some may not be permitted.

There are innumerable other factors which can contribute to our dietary choices. The point here is that it's really common to blame ourselves or our lack of willpower when it comes to our dietary choices, but acknowledging that there are many other influences can be helpful in trying to challenge and change some of them when thinking about your diet and lifestyle goals.

In this chapter we've looked at the individual impact of each dietary component on the immune system and overall health. However, it's also important to note that evidence has shown that the combination of high-salt, high-sugar and high saturated fat intakes in the diet may have a far more damaging impact on the increased risk of chronic inflammatory conditions than each component in isolation. It's also believed that the overconsumption of these dietary components commonly occurs alongside a limited intake of fibre. The combination of an overconsumption of these components plus a low fibre intake may have a negative effect on the gut microbiota. Moreover, in recent years this dietary pattern has become a more significant area of interest in relation to chronic inflammatory diseases such as inflammatory bowel diseases, ulcerative colitis and asthma. As we will explore in Chapter 8, this dietary pattern is often closely associated with the western diet, which is also characterised by large intakes of refined grains, minimal consumption of fruit and vegetables and excess alcohol intake.

In this chapter I've outlined a number of dietary components that when consumed in excess can negatively affect your immunity and general wellbeing. Of course, making the suggested changes to all of these dietary aspects may not feel relevant or necessary to you. Therefore, I recommend looking at your own diet and assessing which of these components you feel you can make changes to.

As I've already suggested, taking an approach to limiting some foods can be far more effective and sustainable in the long term than trying to eliminate them altogether. Additionally, finding the balance may be more beneficial than trying to remove certain dietary components completely. Remember we do need some sugar and salt in the diet to be able to function optimally. This isn't about getting hung up on every ingredient in your food; it's about becoming more aware of your overall diet and the key components which may be influencing your immune health. Dietary change should be a long-term process, so it's OK if it takes a while to work on the points outlined in this chapter.

Finally, remember that it's far more effective in the long run to focus on the reduction of one dietary aspect at a time rather than attempting to drastically reduce salt, sugar and unhealthy fats at the same time.

Summary Points

- High intakes of salt, sugar and saturated fat have been associated with impaired immune function.
- Blood glucose regulation is key in supporting the health of the immune system. Impaired blood glucose regulation can contribute to damaged immune cells and an increase in inflammation.
- Consuming artificial sweeteners in high amounts can have direct and indirect effects on the immune system, through their role in manipulation of the immune cells, their contribution to dysbiosis in the gut and increased risk of inflammation.
- Animal studies have found that regular intakes of food additives – even at low doses – can have adverse effects including inflammation, an increased risk of dysbiosis in the gut and adaptations to appetite regulatory hormones.

CHAPTER 8

Autoimmunity and Dietary Patterns Associated with Autoimmune Conditions

Autoimmunity Explained

Autoimmunity occurs when antibodies or lymphocytes target the healthy cells of the body rather than targeting foreign pathogens. The adaptive immune system is predominantly responsible for autoimmune reactions. An autoimmune reaction occurs when self-antigens (substances which have an internal origin) are identified by the immune system as potential threats. As a result, an immune response can be activated. This process can negatively impact the normal function of the body, depending on which cells are being targeted. A few common examples of autoimmune conditions include inflammatory bowel disease, Hashimoto's disease (a disease of the thyroid), multiple sclerosis and rheumatoid arthritis.

An autoimmune response can be either systemic (a response which occurs across the entire body) or more targeted to a specific site. Examples of targeted immune responses include type 1 diabetes, where the pancreas is attacked, and Hashimoto's disease, where the thyroid is the primary suspect and consequently becomes targeted too.

Factors affecting the development of an autoimmune disease

The triggers for autoimmune diseases are not yet fully understood. However, it's thought that a previous infection, diet and environment can all play a role. Some autoimmune conditions can also be related to a genetic susceptibility, which can increase the likelihood of developing the condition.

For example, multiple sclerosis is well known for its genetic links, although genes alone aren't the sole predetermining factor in developing the disease. Lupus is another autoimmune condition which has strong genetic links. These links are more prevalent in African American and Hispanic populations.

In addition to genes, sex can also influence the risk of autoimmune disease. We know that women are much more likely to develop an autoimmune disease compared to men and this is likely due to their higher levels of oestrogen and progesterone.

Many autoimmune conditions present a variety of similar initial symptoms. Muscle and joint soreness, fatigue, numbness in the hands and feet, brain fog, fever and skin rashes are among the most common early symptoms. However, autoimmune diseases such as inflammatory bowel disease will also produce gastrointestinal symptoms such as changes in bowel movement, blood in stools, cramping, diarrhoea, bloating and gastrointestinal discomfort.

Concerningly, the incidence of autoimmunity in the modern

world is drastically increasing. It's thought that our modern lifestyles, diets and potentially our environment are all playing a role in the prevalence of autoimmune conditions.

Could the Western Diet Be Contributing to an Increased Risk of Autoimmune Conditions?

After the agricultural revolution, farming methods improved the availability of whole foods such as meats, produce, grains and pulses. However, over the last fifty years or so, western diets have evolved once again and, as we saw in the previous chapter, have become far more processed and much higher in sugar and artificial ingredients. The correlation between this change in our diets and the rise in autoimmunity has piqued interest in the role that our diet can play on the development of these conditions.

The modern western diet is one which is characterised as being high in salt, saturated fats, trans fats, sugars and artificial food additives. In the previous chapter we explored each of these in the context of their individual influences on immune health and inflammation. However, we also need to consider if the combination of these dietary components in consistently high intakes could be a recipe for the development of an autoimmune condition.

Let's look at the most concerning dietary pattern: the western diet.

The western diet is subject to drastic overprocessing, often of foods that would otherwise be nutritious ingredients. Modern industrial processing methods result in an array of foods which no longer resemble their original form.

For example, the cacao bean is an ingredient which has been

consumed for over four thousand years. In its most minimally processed form it has been associated with a multitude of health benefits and nutritious properties. However, the 'westernisation' of the cacao bean has led to it becoming hugely overprocessed. When combined with a variety of added ingredients such as sugars, fats, trans fats and artificial additives it becomes unrecognisable from its original form. This overprocessed form, known as chocolate, has become a major product in the western diet.

The western diet has also been associated with an increased risk of intestinal permeability, obesity and low-grade chronic inflammation, all of which are major contributors to the disruption of the immune system and the increased risk of autoimmune conditions. The lack of fibre from fruits, vegetables, nuts, seeds and wholegrains is also thought to impair the function of the gut microbiome and the intestinal mucosal layer, which is integral to immune health. Furthermore, the disruption to the gut and increases in intestinal permeability can contribute to malabsorption. Malabsorption occurs when the gut is unable to sufficiently absorb the nutrients from our foods. What this means is that nutrients which *are* being consumed may not be having the desired effect of supporting the immune function and general physiological function. Since autoimmune conditions can be exacerbated by nutrient deficiencies, the role of malabsorption is one which should always be considered in cases of autoimmunity.

Moreover, the typical western diet is partly responsible for causing regular blood glucose spikes due to the prevalence of high-sugar foods. As we've explored in the previous chapter, consistent blood sugar spikes can contribute to an increase in low-grade, systemic inflammation and the development of non-communicable diseases and autoimmune conditions.

As well as the diet itself, the western lifestyle may also be playing a perpetuating role in the development of autoimmune conditions. When you consider that we are now living with excessive exposure to air pollution, reduced physical activity, reduced exposure to microbial infections and high levels of stress, it's no surprise that it's thought that all of these factors can play a role in the development of autoimmune conditions. As we have seen in previous chapters, there are plenty of practical ways we can improve our diets to optimise immune health, but the above is a reminder that when it comes to strengthening our immune system, we should be prioritising not only our diets but our lifestyle behaviours too.

Can the Mediterranean Diet Play a Role in Reducing the Risk of Autoimmune Conditions?

Evidently the picture which is painted in relation to the western diet and lifestyle and the associated risk of autoimmune conditions is fairly alarming. So how can we address this?

The answer may be in the Mediterranean diet. The Mediterranean diet is one which is characterised as a diet based on whole foods such as fruits, vegetables, nuts, seeds, wholegrains, healthy fats (with the primary source being olive oil) and moderate intakes of high-quality dairy, eggs, fish and poultry. This dietary pattern looks far more similar to the one which we consumed as a result of the agricultural revolution, before the industrial revolution. It is also one which has long been associated with a whole host of favourable health outcomes. The Mediterranean diet has been universally deemed to be one of the most protective and supportive diets for immune health.

It's higher in polyunsaturated fats and is typically lower in omega-6 than the western diet. As previously discussed, higher intakes of omega-3 and lower intakes of omega-6 can favour a more anti-inflammatory state. This dietary pattern is also higher in fibre due to the significant contributions from whole plant foods. Fibre can help to promote T-cell regulation by helping to protect the beneficial microbes in the gut and supporting the production of short-chain fatty acids. The Mediterranean diet is also significantly higher in polyphenols than the western diet, which further helps to protect the integrity of the gut microbes and promotes antioxidative benefits.

In addition to the general beneficial and protective mechanisms of the Mediterranean diet on reducing inflammation and supporting immune health, it's also been associated with benefits in a wide range of specific autoimmune conditions. Moreover, it's significantly associated with a reduction in the risk of coronary heart disease and mortality relating to coronary heart disease, as well as diseases that often occur alongside coronary heart disease. The PREDIMED study, one of the largest studies to date, assessed the role of the Mediterranean diet on cardiovascular disease risk. The study assessed over seven thousand individuals, and the findings showed that a Mediterranean diet high in healthy fats in the form of either extra virgin olive oil or nuts produced a 30 per cent reduction in cardiovascular disease risk when compared to a low-fat diet. The study also demonstrated that the Mediterranean diet reduced the risks of metabolic syndrome, diabetes, hypertension (high blood pressure), oxidative stress and vascular inflammation. Evidently, the type of fats within the diet appears to have an important role in moderating inflammation.

It's also thought that these protective mechanisms are

associated with the anti-inflammatory effects on the vascular wall, lower levels of oxidative stress and a reduction in endothelial dysfunction. Endothelial dysfunction is a common type of coronary artery disease which can occur when the health status of the inner lining of the arteries is compromised. These effects also contribute to a reduction in the risk of atherosclerosis, a disease which causes a narrowing of the arteries.

One study assessed the impact of the Mediterranean diet on rheumatoid arthritis. Participants with a high adherence to the diet showed significant reductions in the inflammatory biomarker C-reactive protein (CRP) and the symptoms of the disease when compared to participants with a moderate to low adherence. Those with high adherence to the Mediterranean diet also presented positive alterations to the gut microbiome. This suggests that the Mediterranean diet may play a role in lowering inflammation derived from rheumatoid arthritis.

There is also promising evidence on the role of the Mediterranean diet in reducing the risks of neurological disorders such as Alzheimer's disease. While this appears positive, further research is required.

All things considered, the evidence displays a strong link between the role of the Mediterranean diet in supporting immune health and reducing the risks of autoimmune diseases. The Mediterranean diet encompasses a wide range of nutritional components required to support immune health and general wellbeing. Therefore, it makes sense to try to incorporate some of the whole-food principles of the Mediterranean diet into our own lives in order to support our health.

How Safe Are Ketogenic and Low-Carbohydrate Diets When It Comes to Autoimmune Diseases?

The ketogenic diet has become one of the most widely searched diets on the internet. Along with low-carbohydrate diets, it's often hailed as the diet to end all diets when it comes to weight management.

The ketogenic diet is a very low-carb, high-fat diet, and was originally designed in the early 1900s to support the management of epilepsy in children. In clinical settings a true ketogenic diet is one that is meticulously calculated and accounts for every gram of fat and carbohydrate. A true ketogenic diet is one which consists of around 70–80 per cent healthy fats and the remainder from a specifically calculated combination of carbohydrates and proteins. Today, however, those commonly following a non-medical ketogenic diet are typically referring to a less meticulously calculated low-carbohydrate diet which involves the significant restriction of the consumption of carbohydrates from sugars, wholegrains, beans, pulses, fruits and vegetables.

For many individuals it can be a very effective method for short-term weight loss. When it comes to inflammation, there is some evidence to suggest that reducing obesity can help to lower the risk of chronic low-grade systemic inflammation. However, due to its highly restrictive framework, maintaining a diet of this nature for a prolonged period of time can be incredibly challenging from a physical, mental and social perspective. As a result, many people are unable to maintain this restrictive diet and, consequently, there is a high risk of regaining any weight lost when they return to their original diet. Additionally, the diet can pose risks of nutrient deficiencies and impaired gut health due to low fibre intakes. Therefore, it's not one which I would encourage you to adopt as a mechanism for weight loss. However, in the interests of science, the mechanisms which can explain any weight loss include blood glucose control, which in turn can help to manage sugar cravings and appetite regulation; an increase in the satiety hormone GLP-1 from protein and fats, which may contribute to a lower total energy intake; reduced water storage; and an increase in gluconeogenesis (an endogenous process which increases glucose production).

Aside from its effect on weight management, what else do we know about the role of the ketogenic diet and other very low-carb diets in autoimmune conditions?

Some research suggests that low-carbohydrate and ketogenic diets may play a significant role in blood glucose management and insulin resistance in diabetic patients. Managing blood sugar control and improving insulin sensitivity can contribute to minimising insulin-derived inflammation.

Furthermore, very low-carbohydrate and ketogenic diets can induce the production of ketone bodies such as acetoacetate, acetone and beta-hydroxybutyric acid. Ketone bodies are an alternative source of fuel that can be used when glucose levels are low. Some research suggests that ketone bodies may induce anti-inflammatory effects, which can help to promote immune function. However, these diets do pose risks for those with diabetes and shouldn't be adopted without the supervision of a healthcare professional. This is particularly important as these diets may also increase the risk of hypoglycaemia, particularly in individuals using insulin as a management tool.

What's more, the terms ketogenic diet, very low-carbohydrate diet and low-carbohydrate diet are often used interchangeably, although they do vary in nature. As highlighted, the ketogenic diet is not just about drastically reducing carbohydrates, it also encompasses the significant contribution of fats in the diet. A low-carbohydrate diet is one which predominantly limits carbohydrates in the diet and replaces them with either fats or protein. There are no set guidelines as to what constitutes a low-carbohydrate or a very low-carbohydrate diet but, typically, a low-carbohydrate diet consists of 50–100g of carbohydrates per day and a very low-carbohydrate diet is one which promotes less than 50g of carbohydrates per day. Unfortunately, the literature too often refers to the terms low-carbohydrate and ketogenic interchangeably, which contributes to what appears to be contradictory results within the research.

As a result, there are some significant conflicts within the research around the role of ketogenic diets, low-carbohydrate diets and very low-carbohydrate diets on the management of a wide range of autoimmune conditions, including inflammatory bowel disease, Alzheimer's disease, Parkinson's disease, type 1 diabetes and multiple sclerosis. Consequently, I'm not in a position to recommend these diets as a management tool. Additionally, it's crucial to note that the research is often conducted on already diagnosed animals and individuals and therefore this does not accurately indicate the role these diets can have on reducing the risk.

Furthermore, when it comes to putting this literature into practice it can be challenging as often the literature fails to distinguish between the different dietary sources of carbohydrates; consequently, we can question whether the benefits found in some of the research are as a result of totally reducing carbohydrate consumption or as a result of lowering intakes of ultra-processed foods and those high in refined sugars. Further research into the sources of carbohydrates in these diets may help us to uncover more definitive answers within this space. Furthermore, it's important to note that very low-carbohydrate diets or ketogenic diets can cause a wide range of side effects such as fatigue, low mood and irritability, headaches, nausea, changes in bowel movements and an increased risk of nutrient deficiencies. Additionally, due to their restrictive nature, they may also pose a risk of a poor gut microbiome.

Dietary patterns may be more helpful in managing the risk of autoimmune conditions than single-nutrient focuses. This is due to the fact that dietary patterns consider the effect of the omega-3 to omega-6 ratios, nutrient interactions and the total combined effects of high intakes of saturated fats, trans fats, sugars and salt. The evidence clearly highlights a strong link between the western diet and lifestyle and an increased risk of autoimmune conditions. Similarly, the research suggests that the Mediterranean diet may play a protective role, helping to lower the risk of autoimmune conditions. However, the effects of the ketogenic diet, low-carbohydrate diets and very low-carbohydrate diets on immune function remain a topic of controversy and their long-term safety remains unknown.

Overall, consuming a dietary pattern that looks more similar to the Mediterranean diet than the western one may be beneficial to supporting health and reducing the risks of autoimmune conditions in the long term. Incorporating some of the principles of the Mediterranean diet is very much aligned with the advice presented throughout the book. As a starting point, try to ensure you're focusing on at least one of the following: consuming one to two portions of oily fish per week (or a daily portion of a source of plant-based omega-3), adding more vegetables to your meals, incorporating nuts and good-quality dairy products into your snacks and limiting your consumption of ultra-processed snacks and fried foods.

Summary Points

- Autoimmunity occurs when antibodies or lymphocytes target the healthy cells of the body rather than foreign pathogens.
- The incidences of autoimmune conditions in the western world are increasing drastically and it's believed that the combination of the western diet and lifestyle is contributing enormously to this increase.
- The western diet is typically high in sugar, salt and fat and the combination of these dietary components lends itself to a more proinflammatory state.
- Evidence suggests that the Mediterranean diet is associated with a significantly reduced risk of chronic inflammatory conditions such as cardiovascular disease, diabetes, atherosclerosis and rheumatoid arthritis.
- Evidence around the use of low-carbohydrate diets and the ketogenic diet to reduce the risk or support the management of autoimmune conditions is not yet fully conclusive. Additionally, the long-term implications of following a very low-carbohydrate diet are not yet fully understood.
- Dietary patterns can be a great way to assess the role of diet on immune health and long-term wellbeing.

CHAPTER 9

Lifestyle Factors Affecting Immune Function

So far we've looked at the role of nutrition and diet in supporting a healthy immune system, but it isn't just the food we're putting into our bodies that we need to consider – other lifestyle factors can be crucial when it comes to optimising your immune health.

Dietary and lifestyle habits can vary hugely from person to person and there are multiple causes which influence our behaviours and how we live and eat on a day-to-day basis. Our childhood and upbringing contributes to a significant aspect of who we are today. In addition, our environment, genetics, familial history, social engagements, economic status, religious and political beliefs, job roles, psychological states, gut microbiome, age and gender are also just some of the many factors that contribute to our individual differences and lifestyles on any given day. In this chapter, I'll walk you through some of the most common lifestyle behaviours that can influence our immune system in both positive and adverse ways. It's OK if not all these factors feel relatable. Although, if there are a few which resonate with you then these are the habits that I recommend you focus on. We can't control every external influence on our immunity, but if you feel you can make micro changes or you can control certain habits, then use that motivation and the information provided to start making your changes today.

The Importance of Balance

When it comes to thinking about your lifestyle, it doesn't have to be an all-or-nothing approach. As you read on you'll see that there are habits presented in this chapter which encourage you to strike a balance between your psychological, physical and social wellbeing, although I will be largely focusing on your physical wellbeing and more specifically the immune system. As ever, balance is key. You might feel that consuming a few pints in the pub on a weekend adds enough fuel to your psychological and social wellbeing to outweigh the negative implications for your immune health. However, if you're hitting the pub multiple times a week for more than one or two then you may want to recognise how the balance is probably tipping too far towards social wellbeing. So what are the lifestyle factors that can impact our immune system?

Am I Sleeping Enough?

Despite the fact that we should be spending over 30 per cent of our lives asleep, sleep has previously often been viewed as an inconvenient exercise designed to clear that familiar tired feeling. However, in more recent years it's become clear that the role of sleep goes far beyond reducing tiredness and fatigue. In fact, it's one of the most important behaviours for optimal health that we engage in. Some have even suggested that sleep may be a greater predictor of long-term health than diet and exercise combined. Consequently, the interest and research into the topic of sleep has climbed the priority ladder and we're really starting to understand the benefits of sleep on our long-term wellbeing. Sleep has a variety of purposes and affects multiple aspects of our health. Not only does it have numerous neurological benefits, immune health benefits, memory consolidation and metabolic benefits, it can also impact our day-to-day behaviours.

If we take science out of the picture for a moment, it's no surprise that sleep plays a critical role in our health and, more specifically, our immune function. Many of us may be familiar with going through a period of ill health following an intense period of lack of sleep.

During sleep, the body works to support the normal function of the immune system. Although when we've fallen ill to an unwanted intruder, sleep becomes even more important as it can help to support the immune response and improve recovery. This can help to explain why we sleep more during periods of ill health. It's also been associated with benefits to immune memory, which is particularly important in the adaptive immune system. Sleep can help to support antibody production and protect against the same intruders in the future. Even when the immune system is not perceived to be 'under attack', it's still constantly working in the background. The period of sleep is a critical time to focus on the production and activity of the immune cells; furthermore, sleep deprivation has been shown to alter the antibody response to certain vaccines and thus can impact the effectiveness of immunisation strategies.

Multiple studies have been shown to support these findings, including one study that assessed the sleep patterns of individuals over a period of fourteen days. The researchers found that individuals who slept less than seven hours per night were three times more likely to catch a common cold when compared to those who slept more than eight hours per night. These findings go to show how even such small adjustments to our sleep may have a significant impact on our immunity.

Furthermore, the relationship between sleep and immunity appears to be a bidirectional one: not only does sleep positively support the functions of the immune cells but specific cytokines, namely interleukin-1 and interleukin-6, have been shown to help support the regulation of our sleep. Adequate sleep has been associated with improved immune function, better response to vaccines, reduced illness and lower incidences of allergic episodes. Generally, we should be aiming for around seven to nine hours of sleep per night.

Impaired sleep can also alter other aspects of our health, which may directly and indirectly affect our immune system. For example, evidence has shown that even one night of sleep deprivation (sleeping four hours per night) can increase levels of the hunger hormone ghrelin and reduce levels of the satiety hormone leptin. This combination is a driver for increased appetite in which we would require more food to feel the same level of fullness as we would following a regular night of sleep. In addition, poor sleep can contribute to significant increases in the desire for high-sugar, high-fat foods which, as we've seen, can also have negative effects on immune cell function when regularly overconsumed. As a one-off, this mechanism is unlikely to cause harm; however, if sleep deprivation is a recurring issue, the overconsumption of these types of foods can begin to have a more substantial effect by increasing the risk of impaired immune health. Furthermore, sleep deprivation can contribute to an excessive reliance on caffeine, alcohol and drugs, which consequently can impact the status of the immune cells too.

Since there are a very small minority of people who can survive on less than seven hours of sleep, you might be wondering how you know if you're getting adequate amounts of sleep. Tuning in to your physiological and psychological cues can answer this quite simply. If you're unsure, try answering the following questions:

- Are you struggling to wake up in the morning?
- Do you feel constantly tired?
- Are you waking up feeling far from refreshed?
- Are you struggling to concentrate throughout the day?
- Are you relying on caffeine to provide you with energy to see you through the day?

If the answer to many of these questions is yes, then your sleep quality or quantity may not be as optimal as it should be.

In a world of micro-stresses the struggle with falling asleep is far too common. Therefore, the following behaviours can really help to optimise your night-time routine, which in turn can give you a better chance of a higher quality of sleep:

- **Avoid caffeine after 2pm.** Caffeine has a half-life of six hours, which means that if you're consuming a coffee at 4pm to see you through the rest of the day, by 10pm half of the caffeine is still circulating in your bloodstream. Caffeine can be problematic as it blocks the neurotransmitters adenosine and GABA, both of which play a role in making you feel calm and sleepy, ready to hit the pillow. Consequently, if they're not being secreted or utilised you'll be feeling more wired than tired. Try switching your 4pm coffee to a herbal tea, a decaffeinated option or hot water with fresh mint.

- **Avoid bright lights or screens in the hour before bed.** Bright light and blue lights emitted from screens can impair the production and absorption of the sleep hormone melatonin. Where possible try to dim the lights and avoid spending time on your emails, watching TV or scrolling social media. If you simply can't avoid screens in the evening then you may want to invest in a pair of blue-light-blocking glasses or a blue-light screen protector, both of which can help to reduce the exposure to blue light.

- **Avoid eating a large meal too late in the evening.** Consuming a large meal before going to bed can cause a disruption to the production and absorption of melatonin, which is secreted and absorbed in the gut. If your body is prioritising digesting your large meal it's less effective at secreting and absorbing the melatonin. Additionally, digesting a large meal drives an increase in core body temperature, which conflicts with the need for a drop in core body temperature for optimum sleep. If you are eating late in the evening try opting for a lighter meal such as a bowl of soup, an omelette or a small bowl of porridge. In such cases you may wish to have a larger meal at lunch to ensure you're providing yourself with enough energy and micronutrients to support your nutritional needs.

Shift work

Shift work can have an effect on our immune system. It is classified as working hours which fall outside of the traditional 9am–5pm working routine. Shift workers may work through the very early hours, late evenings, through the night, or even have to juggle the challenges of rotating shifts. Consequently, sleep deprivation is common among shift workers as they're constantly having to fight against their internal biological clock, light exposure and their own sleep–wake patterns. Evidence has shown that shift work can alter varying factors within the immune system and the productivity of both the innate and adaptive immune cells. As a result, shift workers may be at a greater risk of infection or reduced immune function in response to these factors and as a result of sleep disruption. For many, the lifestyle of shift work may not necessarily be a choice and therefore, much like other dietary and lifestyle factors, it's important that you work within your circumstances. For those who are working shifts, trying to have as much routine with your sleep as possible can help to moderate some of these effects. Additionally, while it can be tempting to consume high-sugar, high-fat foods and caffeinated drinks throughout the night, trying to have two main meals either side of your shift with a high-protein snack in between can help to manage blood sugar levels, energy and overall wellbeing.

Is OK to Have My Coffee in the Morning?

Many of us are searching for that caffeine hit in the morning and, as a result, it's become a common routine to reach for that first mug of coffee as we open our eyes. Caffeine is one of the most abused psychoactive drugs in the world and it's a social and cultural habit which we've adopted worldwide. Although coffee is one of the most common sources of caffeine it's also found in many other products such as tea, chocolate, energy drinks and medications. The maximum recommended intake for healthy adults in the UK is 400 milligrams per day. This equates to around four cups of instant coffee or two cups of barista-made coffee. Be aware that caffeine contents from coffees bought on the go can vary drastically. It's also important to note that this is a maximum recommended intake rather than a target and for many people this amount of caffeine would be considered too much.

Caffeine is absorbed in the small intestine relatively quickly, with an average absorption time of 30–45 minutes, although absorption is slowed by the presence of food. The relationship between caffeine, our health and our immune function is a complex and multidirectional one. Results of research into the benefits and detrimental impacts of caffeine vary greatly. Although, our genes can play a significant role in how we metabolise caffeine and therefore the genetic influence (which is often not accounted for in the research around caffeine) may help to explain the conflicting findings. There are two main genes which can influence the metabolism of caffeine: CYPA1A2 and ADORA2A. Variations in these genes can affect whether we metabolise caffeine quickly or slowly. Currently there's no research to demonstrate how the differences in these genes can impact the influence of caffeine on our health and – more specifically – the immune system. Consequently, the body of the evidence largely looks at caffeine independent of genetic influence, although this is definitely an area in which we require further research.

In addition to the genetic influence on caffeine metabolism, dosages can also contribute to the multitude of effects which caffeine can have on our wellbeing. Single high doses of 300 milligrams or more have been shown to have adverse effects, such as insomnia, redness and flushing, gastrointestinal distress, muscle tremors (otherwise known as the shakes) and tachycardia (a significant increase in heart rate).

Conversely, some evidence has shown that moderate tea and coffee consumption may contribute to reducing the risk of some neurodegenerative diseases such as Alzheimer's disease and Parkinson's disease. It's thought that the antioxidants in coffee can help to reduce oxidative stress which may be one of the contributing risk factors in neurodegenerative diseases. However, it's important to note that the causes of these diseases are often multifactorial and therefore more research is required. Furthermore, these antioxidative effects may also contribute to a reduced risk of skin damage when the caffeine is consumed in the form of coffee. However, we require far more research to understand whether it's the caffeine or other plant compounds present in tea and coffee which may induce these beneficial effects.

Contrarily, caffeine has been found to negatively affect individuals with diagnosed gastrointestinal disorders as it can increase the production of hydrochloric acid and gastric acid, which in excess can reinforce inflammation of the gut lining. Furthermore, there may also be a correlation between a higher caffeine consumption and a greater risk of some respiratory disorders such as chronic obstructive pulmonary disorder (COPD) in those who are prone to these disorders.

It is clear, therefore, that the research around caffeine presents multiple findings as to its effects on immune function and disease risk. Ultimately the effects of caffeine on our overall health and immune function are hugely complex and whether the impact is beneficial or detrimental depends on the individual, type, dose and timing. Despite the array of evidence we currently have, further research is required to fully understand the genetic influence, the mechanisms and the components of caffeine which are eliciting these effects.

For now, the best way to assess how well caffeine sits with you is to do your own social experiment. Try to acknowledge whether it has a positive or negative effect on your wellbeing. Does it leave you feeling jittery, anxious or unable to sleep? If the answer is yes, then you may want to consider cutting back on your caffeine consumption or reassessing the time of day you're consuming it. Reducing caffeine intake doesn't have to mean removing it entirely; cutting back can be as simple as:

- Switching your afternoon coffee for a herbal tea or a decaffeinated option.
- Limiting the amount of chocolate you're consuming. This is particularly key if you're highly sensitive to caffeine.
- Enjoying a decaffeinated tea or coffee every other morning.
- Switching to lower caffeine options such as matcha or green tea.
- Consuming your coffee with food. (Although do be aware that the tannins in tea and coffee can inhibit the absorption of some nutrients such as iron and zinc and some medicines too. Try to avoid consuming these drinks with foods such as oats, green leafy vegetables, nuts and wholegrains.)

Can I Drink in Moderation?

The overconsumption of alcohol is a systemic issue within our society as alcohol plays a central role in far too many social, cultural and sporting events in the UK. Despite the rise in sobriety and the sober curious movement, we're still seeing a spike in alcohol-related hospital admissions. NHS data shows there were 280,000 alcohol-related hospital admissions in 2019/2020. These figures were up by 2 per cent compared to the previous year. The lack of alcohol regulation and education around the risks and adverse effects of overconsumption are significant contributing factors to these statistics.

Evidence has shown that excessive alcohol consumption can have detrimental effects on our overall wellbeing and our immune system. High intakes of alcohol have been associated with an increased risk of immune-related conditions and acute respiratory stress syndromes. Furthermore, a regular large consumption of alcohol can also contribute to an increased risk of alcoholic liver disease and some cancers. Research has also found that excessive alcohol consumption can increase the recovery time in response to diseases and infections as well as slowing down wound healing.

The mechanisms behind these effects on the immune function include damage to essential organs and tissues, a weakening of the defence mechanisms in both the innate and adaptive immune systems and an increase in systemic inflammation. High levels of systemic inflammation may impair the body's ability to maintain immune homeostasis. In addition, alcohol can have detrimental effects on the gut microbiome as it contributes to a rise in pathogenic bacteria, impaired barrier function and damaged gut mucosa.

A permeable gut barrier can enable bacteria to pass through the gut into the bloodstream. This can be problematic as the bacteria (even the beneficial microbes) can cause increased inflammation in the liver, which causes a greater risk of alcoholic liver disease.

Furthermore, alcohol may also contribute to respiratory-related diseases as it's been shown to impair the behaviours of the immune cells within the upper and lower airways in the lungs. In addition to the direct impact that alcohol may have on our immune cell function, alcohol consumption may also contribute to impairing the effectiveness of the response to some vaccines.

Alongside these detrimental effects on immunity, regular alcohol consumption can inhibit the body from working efficiently to maintain normal physiological function. This is because alcohol metabolism can be immensely taxing on our nutritional status and the removal of the poison ethanol can take priority. This means that alcohol metabolism requires excess micronutrients which may contribute to the depletion of nutrients required for other physiological processes.

Striking a balance between enjoying a glass of wine and consuming alcohol in excess has become more and more challenging as our society often normalises the overconsumption of alcohol. However, even acute binge drinking such as consuming just one too many pints or G&Ts on a Saturday night may contribute to impairing our immune health. Let's face it, many of us (myself included) enjoy a glass of rosé in the sun or a rich red by the fire in the winter months. Yet failing to manage our intake and engaging in antisocial drinking or even socially excessive drinking behaviours are detrimental to supporting our immune health and long-term wellbeing. The UK government recommends consuming no more than fourteen units per week for both men and women. In practice this looks like six pints of beer, six small glasses of wine or fourteen single measures of a spirit. These guidelines often surprise people when they start to put into context their weekly alcohol consumption. However, it's important not to instil fear, while still being able to educate, encourage and influence a significant change in our society's attitude towards alcohol.

Fortunately, there are many measures which we can take to help limit or cut down on our alcohol consumption. Try to ensure you're having at least three to four alcohol-free days per week, although avoiding overconsumption on the days you are drinking is obviously important too. I'm a big advocate for staying hydrated with a glass of water between alcoholic beverages since this can help to support hydration status and reduce your total consumption within a given time frame. Where possible, incorporate sparkling water into drinks such as white or rosé wine to dilute the alcohol and reduce the total amount you're consuming.

Opening up the conversation around reducing alcohol intake can be a good place to start. This can help to reduce the societal stigma associated with not drinking; similarly, switching up activities for your social engagements may also help to reduce your total intake. Going for a walk with a friend rather than a drink or meeting for breakfast as opposed to dinner can also make it easier to cut back on your alcohol consumption.

Cigarette Smoking

According to the Office for National Statistics, in 2021, 13.3 per cent of adults in the UK smoked cigarettes. It's promising that these figures fell between 2019 and 2021, although it's still a significant percentage of the population who are exposing themselves and others (via secondary smoking) to the detrimental impacts of cigarette smoke.

Smoking has long been associated with a significantly increased risk of cancers, inflammatory diseases such as multiple sclerosis and all-cause mortality, but how exactly is it impacting the immune system?

Cigarette smoke contains thousands of chemicals and pollutants, including carbon monoxide, reactive oxygen species, carbon dioxide, reactive nitrogen species and nicotine. These chemicals and pollutants can penetrate the lining of the epithelium and then circulate around the body, in turn increasing the activation of proinflammatory cytokines, the risk of systemic inflammation and many inflammatory-related diseases.

Cigarette smoking has also been shown to negatively influence immune function, as it disrupts both the innate and the adaptive immune cells. The adaptations which occur as a result of chronic cigarette smoking have been associated with chronic inflammatory diseases such as rheumatoid arthritis and COPD, alongside autoimmune conditions such as Crohn's disease, hyperthyroidism, multiple sclerosis, ulcerative colitis and inflammatory bowel disease. Unfortunately, the evidence suggests that both primary and secondary cigarette smoking can negatively influence the function of the immune cells, more specifically the T-helper cells (namely TH17), which are involved in the proinflammatory mechanisms of the immune response, are released in response to smoking-initiated inflammation. Furthermore, evidence demonstrates that exposure to cigarette smoke may contribute to imbalances in the T-reg cells.

Smoking causes damage to DNA and physiological oxidative stress which contributes to chronic inflammation and an increase in the production of free radicals. As we've discussed, elevated levels of free radicals contribute to further damage to the immune cells and other cells in the body.

However, it's thought that not all cigarettes will initiate the same responses. The quality of the cigarettes may contribute to the severity of the effects on immune function and disease risk.

Overall, it's evident that smoking contributes to the weakening of immune cells and prolongs the healing of disease and infection.

There are many reasons as to why people smoke and therefore merely suggesting that you quit smoking would be ignorant, naive and unhelpful on my part. Cigarette smoking is addictive for many individuals, so simply highlighting the effects on the immune system is unlikely to lead to anyone stopping smoking. The desire to quit has to come from within and as part of a genuine drive to improve long-term health.

However, if you are looking to reduce your intake or quit entirely there are a whole host of programmes designed to support your decision. Evidence suggests that nicotine replacements such as gum may not be as detrimental as the inhaling of cigarette smoke on the immune system. Therefore, this may be an alternative for those looking to quit cigarette smoking. It's recommended you seek advice from your GP as a first step. Alternatively, if quitting smoking is not something which appears desirable, feasible or even convincing then assessing other areas of your lifestyle behaviours and dietary choices in helping to moderate the disruptive impacts on immune health and general wellbeing is an excellent place to start.

What Is Stress Doing to Me?

Stress is often the emotion which we use to describe an immense feeling of overwhelm and the inability to cope with the demands placed on us, and as such it commonly has negative connotations. However, the stress response is actually one of the most under-valued, life-saving mechanisms that we have. Back in the caveman era our stress response was activated in response to life-threatening events, such as being chased by a wild animal. In such cases, our so-called fight-or-flight mechanism allowed us to fight or flee the situation in an attempt to save our lives. However, in today's world our stress response is activated multiple times a day in response to numerous micro and major stressors. These can include receiving too many emails and demands at work, traffic, technology malfunctions, financial pressures, family issues, environmental issues and political circumstances. As a result, many of us are no longer benefitting from the original purpose of the stress response – in fact we're seeing the rather negative side to it instead. Unfortunately, given the society we live in today and the extensive pressure we are under to fulfil our daily tasks, pay the bills and keep up to date with an ever-changing environment, many of us are living in an almost constant state of stress. While some individuals may thrive under stress, others may crumble; whatever your response at the time, what we do know is that the long-term implications of living in a persistent state of stress can affect us all in an equally damaging fashion.

There are three types of stress:

- **Physiochemical stress** is experienced as a result of environmental factors such as exposure to pollution and toxins, dietary intakes and inflammation.
- **Psychological stress** is the one which we tend to be more familiar with and which we refer to on a regular basis. This includes the feeling of overwhelm and the anxiety which we often feel as a result of high pressure and stress throughout the day.
- **Physical stress** is the stress which is intentionally exerted on the body, for example as a result of exercise or vaccinations.

In addition to these different types of stress we also have different periods of stress which can have individual effects on the body. Acute stress may actually be beneficial in supporting our immune response, while chronic stress is the type which we want to try to limit or avoid at all costs.

Acute stress, i.e. stress which is experienced for a period of time from a few minutes to a few hours, has been shown to have immune-protective effects. It can help to support immune cell function and the healing process through stimulating the innate and adaptive immune cells. The production of cytokines and white blood cells increase in response to acute stress and consequently can work to support the efficiency of the immune system.

Chronic stress, on the other hand, can have adverse effects. This is when stress occurs for a prolonged period of time. Stress triggers the release of the stress hormones cortisol, epinephrine (also known as adrenaline) and norepinephrine (noradrenaline), which in the short term help to provide energy to cope with the challenge at hand. Yet, over a prolonged period of time, the production of these stress hormones continues and excess levels can contribute to many aspects of ill health. High levels of these stress hormones can affect our health status through impacting factors such as our blood vessels and thus increasing the risk of high blood pressure and coronary heart disease. Additionally, when cortisol levels are continuously high they can contribute to an increased risk of cortisol resistance, which can alter the harmony between inflammatory and anti-inflammatory cytokines. In turn this increases the risk of chronic infection, disease and inflammation.

Furthermore, a chronically high level of stress activates the autonomic nervous system, which communicates with the enteric nervous system (this is the nervous system located in the gastro-intestinal tract). The impact of the stress hormones can disrupt normal gut motility, i.e. the contractions of the muscles within the gut. In addition, these changes can also alter the gut microbes by giving rise to higher levels of pathogenic bacteria. All this can have negative implications for the function of the immune cells.

Another key factor to consider with stress is that high levels of cortisol can increase the desire for high-sugar, high-fat foods. The purpose of this is to dampen down the activity of the hypothalamic-pituitary-adrenal (HPA) axis, which plays a role in the secretion of cortisol. This can explain why when you're stressed and you reach for a bar of chocolate you may automatically feel calmer. I'm not suggesting that this is a good long-term stress solution, but it does help to explain some very common stress-related eating behaviours. Over time, the overconsumption of high-sugar and high-fat foods can equally contribute to inhibiting immune cell function and disturbing homeostasis within the immune system.

Evidently the effects of stress on our overall health and our immune system are vast. While completely eliminating stress is both impossible and undesirable, controlling it to the best of our ability can have powerful benefits for our wellbeing and immunity. Hopefully, you can see how our physiology is hugely interlinked and that the immune system works in conjunction with a whole host of other physiological processes, rather than as a standalone mechanism (which is often how it's portrayed).

Stress reduction techniques

Since stress can have such an impact on not only our psychological wellbeing but also our physiological wellbeing, the impact of stress reduction techniques has become a greater area of interest within the research. The role of mindfulness on our health has become more and more evident and research now shows that engaging in mindfulness strategies can have a significant impact on our immune function too.

Mindfulness meditation is the process in which we can achieve an intentional awareness of a variety of sensations within the body. Engaging in mindfulness activities is associated with a reduction in the concentrations of proinflammatory cytokines. These activities may also reverse some of the negative effects of stress in those with chronically high levels. However, alongside its therapeutic effects, mindfulness can also have protective effects on increasing the concentrations of natural killer cells and B-cells in those who practise regularly.

In addition to mindfulness, engaging in stress-lowering activities on a regular basis can contribute to keeping stress hormones at bay and consequently supporting immune cell function. It's far easier to talk about stress reduction than put it into practice. However, building a few small habits into your daily routine can have wonderous effects on not only your physiological wellbeing but your psychological health too. Pick out one or two of the tips below which you feel would be realistic to incorporate into your daily or weekly routine.

- **Wake up thirty minutes earlier.** This is the perfect time to engage in breathing techniques, sit quietly with a cup of tea or enjoy a short online yoga practice. However, this activity shouldn't mean that you cut your sleep short; instead, try going to bed half an hour earlier in the evening to give you extra time in the morning. If you have children and mornings tend to be rushed, this time can do absolute wonders for your headspace and your approach to the day.

- **Try a gratitude practice or journaling before bed.** Once again this doesn't have to take a long time: spending just five minutes thinking and writing about what you're grateful for from the day or journaling your emotions can help to lower stress levels and over time it can encourage you to think more positively too. On a personal note, I've been keeping a gratitude diary for over six years. It takes me a few minutes in the morning and few minutes in the evening and I can honestly tell you that I think it really changed my perspective on every day. I couldn't recommend it enough.

- **Engage in movement.** We often think about movement in the form of exercise which can entail going to the gym or going for a run but even a few simple stretches in the morning can help to lower stress levels. Additionally, walking outside can help with lowering stress due to the endorphins that we release in response to nature. Where possible try to find some green space or a safe space to walk, even if you've only got five minutes a day.

- **Remind yourself of things you enjoy.** As we get older and our responsibilities grow, it's all too common to fall into the hamster wheel of life where we're so focused on carrying out daily tasks that we forget what's important to us and what makes us happy. Write a list of activities which you enjoy and engage in at least one activity per week to help support stress reduction, your immune health and your psychological wellbeing.

How Does Physical Activity or Exercise Impact My Immunity?

The terms physical activity and exercise are often used interchangeably, although their definitions do vary slightly. Physical activity includes any movement which requires the engagement of skeletal muscle and initiates an increase in heart rate and resting metabolic rate (the amount of energy utilised at rest). This can include walking up the stairs or carrying heavy shopping. Exercise, on the other hand, is a planned physical activity which is carried out at a more intense level and comes with the intention of supporting health or physical fitness. The literature often uses both terms loosely and interchangeably but from here on in we'll be referring to the benefits of exercise, which can include activities carried out at a lower intensity but always with the intention of supporting health and the immune system.

Exercise is regularly celebrated as one of the core pillars of healthy living. It's well understood for its role in supporting a reduced risk of non-communicable diseases such as type 2 diabetes, cardiovascular disease and obesity, all of which are associated with an increase in systemic inflammation.

Participating in regular exercise can positively influence the immune system, although the type and the intensity of the exercise may alter the way in which the immune system responds. Regular exercise increases immunosurveillance and immunocompetence as it can temporarily increase the activity of macrophages and anti-inflammatory cytokines. This means the immune cells are able to react faster and with more specificity in the event of an intruding pathogen.

Exercise also initiates an acute stress response, which, as we've discussed, stimulates the activity of both the innate and adaptive immune cells. In addition to this, engaging in exercise can also promote beneficial antioxidative effects. These effects can work towards neutralising free radicals and lowering oxidative stress, to prevent unwarranted cell death.

The beneficial effects of exercise on immune function can also work in synergy. The collaborative benefits include improvements to the gut microbiome, the direct influence on anti-inflammatory cytokines, the reduction in inflammation and the stimulation of an acute stress response, all of which can be beneficial in supporting the immune response.

Moreover, exercise can help to protect against the detrimental effects of an exposure to dangerous pathogens. For example, experiences from previous pandemics have shown inactive elderly individuals with pre-existing diseases and obesity were more likely to respond worse to the infectious pathogen when compared to active elderly individuals. Exercise can also help with lowering obesity-related adverse immune function. Obesity has long been associated with higher levels of circulating pro-inflammatory cytokines and low-grade systemic inflammation. It's clear that regular exercise can help to reduce the levels of inflammatory cytokines and systemic inflammation. The mechanism behind this may be two-fold: the effects of exercise alone can contribute to lowering inflammation in those with obesity but the role of weight loss *in response to* exercise may also be a contributing factor as to why inflammation decreases for those living with obesity.

We should definitely be using exercise to our advantage, particularly throughout the winter months (where it can be typically more challenging) as it can be a great strategy for helping to ward off winter cold and flu. Animal studies have shown that engaging in intense exercise prior to an infection can help to reduce the intensity of the symptoms and the duration of the infection. This has also been supported with human studies: one assessed 1,002 adults between the ages of eighteen and eighty-five and followed them throughout the twelve weeks of autumn and winter. The researchers found that those who engaged in aerobic exercise for five or more days throughout the week had a 43 per cent reduction in upper respiratory tract infections when compared to sedentary individuals.

The relationship between exercise and the gut microbiome can also impact the immune system. Mice studies have shown that active mice present significant modifications to the gut microbiome when compared to sedentary mice.

The findings from one study showed that exercise positively altered up to 2,510 microbes within the gut. This study controlled for diet and concluded that these findings were independent of the influence of diet on the microbiome. Additional mice studies have shown that exercise can also counteract the negative effects of a high-fat diet on the gut bacteria.

Equally, one study assessed the microbiome of rugby players and compared it to the gut bacteria profiles of healthy control subjects. The rugby players were found to have far greater diversity within their gut microbiome. Although this study failed to control for diet and thus we can't categorically conclude that exercise alone was the sole driver of these differences, this definitely does support the potential role of exercise on improving the diversity of the gut microbes. As we know, an improved gut microbiome profile can support the integrity of the immune system.

Moreover, exercise has also been shown to reduce the transit time of pathogens in the gut and consequently increases the speed of excretion of unwanted pathogens. As a result, this helps to decrease the time in which the unwanted pathogens can interact with the bacteria in the microbiome. This may also be another mechanism for how exercise supports the immune system.

Evidently exercise plays a vital role in improving and supporting our cardiometabolic health, musculoskeletal health and respiratory health and these benefits all also indirectly contribute to maintaining a healthy immune system. Along with the physical benefits of engaging in regular exercise, there are also a whole host of benefits in supporting our psychological wellbeing too, as the reduction in stress that many experience through exercise may also contribute to the benefits of exercise on our immune health.

The recommendations for adults in the UK are to engage in 75 minutes of vigorous exercise or 150 minutes of moderate exercise per week. For some this is an easy target to achieve, while for others it's more difficult as exercise can bring up very contrasting emotions. Some people are instantly taken back to the days where they stood in PE class with that nauseous feeling as they waited to be chosen for the team sport. However, others may see it as an important positive activity in their lives. Often for the individuals who resonate with the former description there can be a hesitance around engaging in exercise or physical activities and consequently many endeavour to avoid it.

On a positive note, exercise doesn't have to look the same for everyone. Engaging in exercise can involve enjoying some gentle movement via an online yoga or Pilates class, getting out for a walk with friends, joining a sports team, attending a dance class or hitting the gym hard if that's more of an appeal. Whether you prefer to exercise alone or enjoy the social aspect of team sports, there is usually something to suit you, it's just about finding the right activity!

Can overexercising harm the immune system?

As with everything, too much of a good thing can be problematic and the same is true when it comes to exercise and the immune system. There are a variety of reasons why too much exercise can negatively impact immune function.

Exercise can be highly demanding and taxing on our physiological health and when carried out to excess with minimal rest it can quickly shift from being a positive acute stressor to a negative chronic stressor. This in turn may contribute to a more chronic inflammatory state. Also, since exercise uses up more of your macro and micronutrients, inadequate refuelling may leave the body depleted of key nutrients required to support immune cell function, which can further contribute to a suppressed immune function. Furthermore, excessive exercise can cause an increased risk of dysbiosis in the gut and permeability of the gut lining, a recipe for impaired immunity.

There has also been some research to suggest that elite athletes are at a greater risk of contracting upper respiratory tract infections. In such cases, symptoms have shown to have a longer-lasting effect in these athletes than those who engage in mild to moderate exercise.

While more research is required into understanding where the sweet spot lies and the exact mechanisms behind the relationship between overexercise and impaired immunity, it's evident that where possible we ought to be engaging in moderate amounts of exercise. For those athletes and individuals who engage in exercise as part of elite sports, exercise will be a vital aspect of their lifestyle. In such cases, optimising their health through adequate dietary support, ample rest where possible and optimal sleep can help to support immunity.

Is Cold Water Therapy Good for Immunity?

As cold water therapy is beginning to gain more and more traction, you may be familiar with the idea. Cold water therapy is the act of submerging the majority of the body in cold water. Despite it being used as a therapy for decades it's only recently that public interest has started to peak. There are many different types of cold water therapy, among them cryotherapy, ice baths, cold showers and cold water swimming. The phenomenon currently boasts multiple health benefits, including supporting mental wellbeing, aiding exercise recovery and supporting immune health via inflammation-reducing mechanisms.

Cold water therapy is believed to work through the physiological and biochemical changes which occur in response to exposure to cold water. Research has shown that the stress and inflammatory responses of regular and well-practised cold water swimmers was far better than those who do not regularly engage in cold water exposure. The suggested mechanisms behind these potential benefits of cold water therapy are a reduction in proinflammatory cytokines, hypoxic stress (low levels of oxygen in the blood) and reactive oxygen species which are produced as a by-product of inflammation. Furthermore, cold water therapy can contribute to short-term vasoconstriction of the blood vessels. This limits the ability of the circulating proinflammatory cytokines. Consequently, this would suggest that cold water therapy may play a significant role in helping to reduce inflammation.

One small-scale study assessed patients with chronic obstructive pulmonary disorder. Participants were assessed for ten weeks, where they had five cold water exposures per week. The results showed a significant increase in lymphocytes, suggesting that cold water therapy can help to support the production of white blood cells – a vital component of the innate immune system.

Moreover, a vast majority of the research conducted on cold water therapy has looked into the effects of cold water therapy on exercise recovery. The evidence suggests that cold water therapy may be beneficial in lowering the acute inflammation which is generated in response to exercise. While the research appears promising in relation to systemic inflammation and supporting the immune function, additional studies are required before we can come to a final conclusion.

Cold water therapy can be a high-risk activity for some individuals and therefore it should be practised in safe environments, with a gradual build-up to the duration of exposure and the temperature of the water. The risk of a cold shock is the most common risk and occurs as a result of a sudden drop in body temperature. The symptoms of a cold shock can include an increase in the stress response, gasping and hyperventilating and an increase in blood pressure. Generally speaking for healthy individuals cold water therapy is deemed safe as long as it's practised responsibly. However, for those with underlying medical conditions, heart problems, the elderly or those at risk of hypothermia it may not be deemed to be safe. If you're interested in exploring cold water therapy, it's recommended to speak to your GP or healthcare professional first. Following this, ensure you're building up your tolerance to cold water gradually, increasing the duration of exposure rather than going in for too long or at a too low temperature initially, as this can be dangerous.

Exposure to Environmental Pollution

Environmental pollutants are one of the greatest challenges to our lifestyle as our exposure to them is often far beyond our control. Unfortunately, air pollution in many urban areas far exceeds the safety limits proposed by the World Health Organization. As a nation, we are slowly working towards better air quality; however, the speed at which we're moving quite simply isn't fast enough. In Chapter 3 we discussed how environmental pollutants can impair the integrity of the gut lining. In the next few paragraphs, I'll expand on this to highlight how they can influence the immune cells too.

It's no secret that excessive exposure to air pollutants can increase the risk of lung disorders, cancers, cardiovascular diseases and all-cause mortality. Thus chronic exposure to environmental pollutants can have a significant negative impact on immune function.

Inhaled pollutants can gather in the macrophages in the lymph nodes located in the lungs. Macrophages that contain pollutants have been shown to lower immune activation and phagocytic activity (phagocytosis is the process in which the immune cells consume the unwanted pathogens). Naturally, the concentration of pollutants in the body increases as we age so, over a prolonged period of time, high exposure to environmental pollutants can alter our immunosurveillance (the ability of the immune cells to look for unwanted pathogens and foreign bodies) and weaken the immune system.

That said, we do require further evidence on how different types of pollutants and the sizes of their particles may impact immune function, yet this worrying mechanism behind the build up of these pollutants highlights our need to work together as a population to make changes to the air quality in our environment.

One of the most researched groups of individuals in this area are firefighters as they are heavily exposed to pollutants and heat. Evidence has shown that firefighters are more likely to display high levels of the inflammatory biomarker C-reactive protein (CRP). CRP indicates levels of inflammation in the body. Firefighters are not alone; there are many other industry roles which put people at greater risk of a compromised immune system as a result of exposure to hazardous waste products, industrial chemicals and environmental pollutants.

It's worth noting, however, that the work of firefighters (and many other similar occupations) is immensely physical, psychologically stressful and requires a pattern of shift work, as well as having a high exposure to the by-products of combusted materials. Therefore, these factors may also play a role in contributing to the increased risk of inflammation associated with the profession.

The impacts of microplastics on immune health is also an area of growing concern as they're present in multiple aspects of our lives. Microplastics are a collection of synthetic particles which are foreign to the immune system. As a result, the immune cells can struggle to remove them from the body. Once in the system, microplastics can release chemicals into the bloodstream, posing an even greater risk to our immune health. In very high levels, these chemicals can contribute to increased oxidative stress, inflammation and damage to the immune cells and the gut microbiota.

As long as we're living in a modern world, completely controlling our exposure to microplastics will remain incredibly challenging. Given that they can be found in many commercial cosmetic products, the air outside, our food and drink and its packaging (with bottled water being one of the most common sources of exposure), managing our exposure is tough.

Despite this, small changes to our behaviours can help to make a difference. Where possible avoid buying drinks (particularly water) in plastic bottles, opt for a glass bottle or carry a reusable one with you. Where possible, try to avoid cosmetic products that contain small beads such as exfoliators and where possible opt for more sustainable and less synthetic clothing too. Finally, avoid buying fruit and vegetables in plastic bags and opt for loose produce where you can. Although these may not seem like drastic changes, over time the benefits can add up and you will be helping to reduce your exposure to microplastics.

Similarly, we may not be able to control the pollutants in the air that we're breathing, yet many of us are able to control smaller exposures to chemicals and pollutants. Try to reconsider the products you're using within your home, for example, the candles you're burning, fires burnt for leisure throughout the winter, barbecue exposure, cleaning and laundry products and the use of fragrances or beauty and wellbeing products containing chemicals.

How Does the Menopause Affect Immunity?

The menopause is a natural part of the female ageing process and is the stage at which women stop producing reproductive hormones. The menopausal period occurs in three phases: the first is the peri-menopause, when the release of sex hormones are on the decline and female menstrual cycles may begin to take a new and more sporadic pattern. The second phase is the menopause and refers to the specific day where a woman has not had a menstrual period for a year. Following this single day, women then enter the post-menopausal stage, where sex hormones are significantly lessened and begin to stabilise.

Often the combination of the menopause and something called immunosenescence can leave post-menopausal women noticing changes to their immune systems. Immunosenescence is the natural impact of ageing on the decline of the immune system and occurs in both women and men. Ageing is related to a significant decline in vaccine response, skeletal muscle function, digestive health and cardiovascular function. However, the menopause has been shown to have more specific implications on the function of the immune cells.

In Chapter 1, we looked at the differences between the function of the male and female immune systems. The strength of the female immune system can be partly attributed to the presence of oestrogen and progesterone. Prior to the menopause oestrogen and progesterone contribute to regulating the function of the immune cells; in particular, oestrogen plays a vital role in protecting against the destruction of B-cells and promoting B-cell formation. Because of this, when oestrogen levels decline there's a significant reduction in the number of B-cells and thus antibody production.

The menopause has also been shown to alter a variety of immune-mediated markers which can highlight the changes that occur as a result of the menopause.

Firstly, there are numerous changes to the vaginal tract acidity levels. This can explain why there is an increased risk of urinary tract infections in post-menopausal women. Furthermore, evidence has shown that post-menopausal women are more prone to an increase in proinflammatory markers. These include higher levels of the cytokines IL-1, IL-6 and TNF alpha. Alongside the decline in B-cell activity, the actions of the natural killer cells also slow. Consequently, this impairs the immune cells' ability to respond to unwanted pathogens. All these changes are driven by the decline in oestrogen.

The menopause may be an inevitable aspect of female physiology but making healthier dietary and lifestyle choices throughout this period can be powerful in ensuring you're setting yourself up for success. Consequently, in the years leading up to the menopause and throughout the period of hormonal fluctuations there are habits which you can engage in to ready yourself.

Ensuring adequate vitamin D status is one of the most important things you can do to support your health at this time. In fact, this should be a non-negotiable for all of us and particularly those entering the menopausal transition. Not only does vitamin D play a vital role in supporting calcium absorption, bone health and mood, all of which can be compromised as a result of the menopause, it's also essential in supporting immune function. Vitamin D deficiency among menopausal women has been associated with an increased risk of susceptibility to infections and autoimmunity.

Adequate vitamin D status has also been shown to increase the production of antibacterial peptides and the autophagic activity of the macrophages. Autophagy is the process that removes and recycles imperfect cells in order to prevent further damage.

Engaging in many of the other healthy habits discussed in this book can also help to promote a healthier menopause. Reducing alcohol consumption, changing smoking habits, engaging in stress-lowering activities and taking regular physical exercise (including resistance-focused or weight-bearing exercises) are all positive strategies for supporting yourself through the menopausal period. Needless to say, improvements in dietary choices and small but sustainable changes can also play a fundamental role in promoting a healthier menopause.

Can Intermittent Fasting Help or Hinder Immunity?

Intermittent fasting is a dietary protocol that has really taken off in the last decade. The body of evidence around intermittent fasting is growing drastically, which means we can make a clearer assessment of the impact of fasting on our health and our immunity.

There are a multitude of patterns which people employ for intermittent fasting protocols. These can include the 16:8 fast, where individuals fast for 16 hours a day and consume all their food within an 8-hour eating window; 5:2 fasts, where calorie intake is significantly restricted to 500 calories on two days a week; and then there are those who take fasting to the extreme and engage in fasts lasting anywhere between 24 and 72 hours. While there are a number of proposed benefits related to intermittent fasting, such as weight management and moderate beneficial effects to the gut microbiome, there may also be some adverse effects.

Intermittent fasting can have negative detrimental effects on those with an eating disorder (or a history of an eating disorder), it can contribute to ruining the social aspect of eating, increase the risk of nutritional deficiencies if adequate nutrients are not consumed within the eating window and it can impact blood glucose regulation in diabetic individuals too. It's also not recommended for those trying to conceive or pregnant women. As it's a relatively new phenomenon, we're still currently unaware of the long-term implications of fasting on our health and wellbeing.

With regard to the role of fasting on the immune system, there may be a sweet spot at which it can be beneficial in supporting immunity. Fasting promotes the process of autophagy, a physiological process which works to engulf and clean up damaged cells and recycle them into molecules that can be used for other mechanisms. Additionally, some of these molecules include key nutrient-rich molecules such as fatty acids and amino acids. If nutritional intakes are low, this is one way in which the body tries to counteract a low nutritional status. However, it will not necessarily entirely replace your requirements. Furthermore, autophagy helps to modulate macrophages, T-cells and B-cells and supports the activity of the natural killer cells. The process of autophagy also plays a key role in the production of antibodies and the release of cytokines.

In addition, intermittent fasting has been shown to increase insulin sensitivity and reduce inflammation, which can help to reduce the risk of type 2 diabetes. It may also often induce a calorie deficit, which is one of the reasons why it contributes to fat loss. A reduction in fat mass can lower proinflammatory cytokines and consequently may further reduce low-grade chronic inflammation.

For some people, fasting in moderation can help to support the immune cells in the gut as it contributes to apoptosis, a process which kills the defenceless immune cells. But when fasting is taken to the extreme, the microbes in the gut look to feed off the mucus of the gut lining and consequently this can increase the risk of permeability.

Evidently there are pros and cons to intermittent fasting and as with all significant changes to your dietary protocols it's always a good idea to seek personalised advice from your healthcare professional to assess whether it is a safe approach for you. Do be aware that a prolonged period of fasting may have adverse effects on your general health and wellbeing, immune function and gut health.

Do Household Pets Help or Hinder the Immune System?

When it comes to the immune system, household pets are an interesting one. The obvious school of thought is that they're an easy transporter of unwanted pathogens into the home. Their behaviours, lack of hygiene awareness and longing to explore every piece of rubbish or dirt they walk past suggests that they would be a constant threat to our immune system. Interestingly, though, household pets can actually have some positive effects on our immune system and our general wellbeing.

Living with household pets is known to help support more positive mental health since their presence can contribute to the secretion of serotonin, the happy hormone. (Admittedly, and as a dog owner myself with first-hand experience, they can also on occasion ramp up those stress hormones.) In addition to this, some household animals such as dogs can also encourage you to get outside and go for daily walks. These walks can not only support your physical wellbeing and immune health but being outdoors and engaging in movement can help to improve your mental health too.

Exposure to household pets can also have a more direct effect on our immune health. A long-term study conducted on 474 children demonstrated that exposure to cats and dogs in the early years significantly reduced the risk of allergies to cats and dogs at the age of six or seven. Additionally, those who were brought up with two or more cats and dogs had a far lower risk of allergies during their childhood. Additional research shows that the early exposure to household pets may also reduce the risk of atopy-related diseases such as asthma and allergic rhinitis. Evidence suggests that exposure to pets, particularly from a young age, can help to diversify the gut microbiome. The increased exposure to pathogens as a result of household pets can support the growth and the development of the adaptive immune system. These benefits extend beyond those pets we typically keep in the home; those who are regularly exposed to farm animals can also reap the same rewards.

These results are promising and suggest that pets can contribute to supporting immune health through a variety of mechanisms. Although it's important to note that for immunocompromised individuals, exposure to household pets can pose significant threats to the immune system.

It's clear how important lifestyle factors are in helping or hindering the immune function. It's common to solely seek out dietary components and nutritional factors to influence the immune system, yet ensuring our lifestyles are aligned with promoting immunity is equally imperative. Hopefully from this chapter you can now see how all aspects of our daily living can impact immunity and general wellbeing. It's reassuring to know that we can really use this information to our advantage: if you think about your morning routine for example, there will be so many opportunities for you to make healthier lifestyle changes in order to support your immunity. Everything from the quality of your sleep, your morning coffee, the temperature of your shower, whether or not you're engaging in physical activity or mindfulness and even the cosmetic products you're using on your skin can all make a difference. As with the dietary advice in this book, I'm not suggesting you overhaul everything all at once, but you may wish to focus on one or two areas of your routine as a starting point for implementing healthier lifestyle habits.

Summary Points

- Many lifestyle factors impact the function of our immune cells. Some of these are more manageable than others, but not all of them are within our control.
- The overconsumption of alcohol and engaging in smoking are two common lifestyle habits that contribute to the degradation of our immune cells. Unfortunately, societal norms are a common driving factor for the maintenance of these habits.
- Stress is a major contributing factor to our overall health and immunity. Long-term significant stress has been shown to contribute to a high risk of chronic systemic inflammation, the production of inflammatory cytokines and degradation of immune cell activity. Engaging in stress-lowering activities can help to promote a healthier immune system.
- Participating in regular moderate physical activity has been associated with a wide range of beneficial immune responses, such as improved immunosurveillance, immunocompetence and the production of anti-inflammatory cytokines.
- Regular exercise can also have positive effects on supporting beneficial microbes within the gut, which can directly support immune cell function.
- Overexercise can have adverse effects on inflammation and the gut microbiome and can lead to an increased risk of infection.

- Cold water therapy has been shown to help reduce exercise-induced acute inflammation but more research into its potential benefits on immune function is needed. Cold water therapy can pose risks and therefore you should always consult a healthcare professional ahead of engaging in cold water therapy.
- Our exposure to environmental pollutants is having a detrimental impact on our immune system and increasing the risk of many lung-related conditions. While we are largely unable to control the particles within the air we're breathing, we can control extra exposure to indoor fires, barbecue smoke and chemical exposure within our homes.
- Throughout the menopause women undergo changes which can contribute to impaired immune cell health and increases in the presence of proinflammatory markers. Engaging in healthy activities and ensuring ample vitamin D status are important aspects of a healthier menopausal transition.
- Intermittent fasting can have pros and cons in terms of supporting our overall health and more specifically the immune system. Engaging in intermittent fasting protocols safely may help to promote autophagy, apoptosis in the gut and reduce low-grade chronic inflammation.
- Having a household pet from a young age can help to reduce the risk of allergies later on in life. Household pets can also support positive mental wellbeing and a more diverse gut microbiome.

CHAPTER 10

Should I Be Taking Supplements?

In the world of nutrition and specifically alongside the topic of immunity, dietary supplements are one of the most popular topics of conversation. Dietary supplements are manufactured nutrients which can be taken to help support nutritional intake. However, they're often far more complicated than simply popping a pill in the morning and, as we're about to explore, the decision to take them should be carefully considered. They're often considered a quick and easy fix, particularly when we're coming down with an illness, so this makes them an interesting area of research. Although, the key question is . . . do we really need supplements? And, if so, what should we be supplementing with? Let's take a deeper look.

My attitude towards nutrition and health has always been that we should take a 'food first' approach. Focusing on whole foods not only provides a multitude of opportunities to seek joy through our meals but also the ability to deliver a constant stream of nourishment to our bodies. Furthermore, in prioritising whole foods over supplements, we gain the advantage of consuming the nutrients which are contained within their co-factors (i.e. their supporting nutrients), which in many cases can help to increase nutrient absorption and bioavailability, essentially the amount of nutrient we can absorb and utilise in the body. The classic term 'you are what you eat' has more recently been recoined to 'you are what you digest', which recognises the importance of bioavailability and accounts for those nutrients that are absorbed and those which are lost throughout the digestion process. When we solely focus on the food consumed we're not accounting for any physiological impairments that can negatively impact absorption and consequently nutritional status. We'll come on to the factors which impact bioavailability later in this chapter.

Another reason to focus on whole foods as opposed to supplements is that whole foods also contain phytochemicals, which are less commonly found in single-nutrient or even multi-nutrient supplements. As we've explored in the previous chapters, phytochemicals have been associated with a multitude of health benefits, such as supporting neurological function, gut health and immune cell function. There are hundreds of phytochemicals but the most common ones include polyphenols, flavanols, fibres, phytosterols and phytoestrogens.

Supplement Considerations

Even with this focus on consuming whole foods, there is absolutely a role for supplements. They can help to protect against nutritional deficiencies, promote optimal health and support the function of the immune system. However, as a society we tend to fall into two camps: the abusers and the underusers.

Ironically, the abusers tend to be those individuals who

don't really need the supplements, as their awareness generally means they're far more likely to be obtaining adequate nutrients through their diet anyway. Conversely, underusers are generally those who would obtain the most benefit from improving their dietary choices and utilising supplements where necessary.

Abusing supplements is an easy habit to slip into as they have become so widespread and accessible. Unlike pharmaceutical drugs, you don't need a prescription from the GP to stock up a supplement cupboard. Despite the common perception that supplements can only do good, they can have adverse effects on our health. For example, taking high-dose supplements can increase the risk of nutrient toxicity, a risk which is rarely posed when nutrients are derived from whole foods.

Water-soluble nutrients cannot be stored in the body and are excreted when consumed in excess. As a result, toxicity isn't as much of a concern with this group of supplements, although some water-soluble nutrients consumed in excess can still induce unfavourable side effects. For example, high doses of vitamin C can induce nausea, vomiting, headaches and gastrointestinal discomfort. On the other hand, fat-soluble vitamins (vitamins A, D, E and K), which can be stored in the body, can pose a more extreme risk of toxicity when they're overconsumed in supplement form.

In some cases, taking high doses of specific nutrients can negate their role entirely. For example, supplementing with very high doses of zinc, which is commonly used to support immune function, can contribute to a suppression in the activity of immune cells, reduce high-density lipoprotein (otherwise known as the good cholesterol) and may also cause a depletion in copper status, as it can inhibit copper absorption from food.

The liver plays a vital role in nutrient metabolism and therefore in addition to the risk of toxicity, consuming unnaturally high doses of individual nutrients can put immense pressure on the liver. When individuals are taking very high doses of a range of nutrients regularly this can increase the risk of liver damage.

In my experience of working with one-to-one clients over the years, I have seen many people who enter my clinic with a lengthy list of supplements that they're taking on a regular basis. Often, these supplement lists are a collection of products which have been recommended to them by friends and family members based on their individual experiences. These supplements might be effective in isolation; however, when taking a large range of supplements, it's not uncommon to double up on nutrients which further increases the risk of nutrient toxicity. For example, if you're taking a single-nutrient supplement such as vitamin C, vitamin D or zinc alongside a multi-nutrient complex such as an immunity complex, a stress support supplement or a general multivitamin, the chances are you're likely to be taking too much of a single nutrient that is present in both.

Another universal issue which occurs as a result of self-prescribing supplements is the potential risk of nutrient–nutrient or drug–nutrient interactions. In some instances, nutrients compete for the same transporters, which are required to absorb and utilise them effectively. As a result, if one nutrient is consistently winning the transporter, the other might be providing little to no benefit. This could be the nutrient which is more favourable in supporting your nutritional needs. Additionally – and more critically – supplements can interact with medications and impair their absorption. For example, vitamin C is well known for interacting with some types of hormonal contraceptives, which can affect the efficiency of some contraceptive pills.

A further consideration for supplementation should be the type of supplement you're taking as not all supplements are equal or are used in the same way. Supplements are available in an assortment of product types, including sprays, liquids, powders, gummies, capsules, tablets and even creams. However, the delivery method can have a significant impact on the bioavailability of these nutrients. What's more, the added ingredients in each product may conflict with supporting optimal health. For example, gummy vitamins are often very high in sugar and therefore generally speaking it's advised not to use these as a method of meeting your nutritional intake. Additionally, many supplement products can contain food additives, artificial binding and anti-caking agents, with some even containing artificial sweeteners. Surprisingly, in spite of some of the risks associated with high-dose supplements and the ease with which they can be purchased, the regulation of the supplement market in the UK is weak, which means that manufacturers are often able to use low-quality ingredients that may not be as accessible to the body. As a result, in some cases, supplements may not have the desired effect if they're not being absorbed or utilised efficiently.

Sprays or liquids can sometimes be better absorbed than capsules or tablets. Although, personal preferences and often the age and capabilities of the individual will guide personal choice on which product and delivery method to use.

Furthermore, the base used in a supplement can also impact its efficiency. Magnesium supplements are a classic example of this as they come in a variety of forms attached to an array of bases, many of which can cause gastrointestinal discomfort in some people, with common side effects including bloating, cramping and diarrhoea. Additionally, some iron supplements can also induce undesirable gastrointestinal symptoms such as constipation and changes in bowel movements. However, iron bisglycinate, which is commonly referred to as gentle iron, can be far gentler on the gut and is typically well absorbed into the bloodstream.

Taking into account all the above, nutrient supplementation should be approached with caution, care and consideration. If you're unsure as to whether or not you should be supplementing always seek personalised advice from your healthcare provider.

When Can Supplements Be Helpful?

When supplement advice is provided via a healthcare professional who has knowledge of your medical background, supplements can be useful. Even marginal nutrient deficiencies can have adverse effects on the immune system and other physiological processes so supplements can help to reduce the risks of deficiency or correct nutrient deficiencies when they occur.

Individuals following a vegetarian or vegan diet can benefit greatly from supplementing with some of the nutrients that are at highest risk of being excluded or limited from these diets. While it is possible to obtain most fundamental nutrients from a vegetarian or vegan diet, there are some which pose a higher risk of deficiency due to the lack of dietary sources or poor absorption rates from plant-based foods. Iron, vitamin B12, vitamin D, omega-3 and iodine are considered some of the higher risk nutrients on these diets. Furthermore, individuals on a medically prescribed diet such as a low residue or keto diet may also be at a greater risk of nutritional deficiencies, due to a decreased variety of foods in the diet.

Nutritional requirements can vary greatly depending on life stage so in some cases obtaining adequate amounts through the diet alone can be challenging. For example, older adults may struggle with consuming the same amount of food as they previously would have, although their nutritional requirements often increase to support the natural process of ageing. Elderly people are also more likely to struggle with absorption and utilisation of nutrients, which can further increase their need for higher intakes.

Pregnancy is another example where nutritional requirements increase significantly, and supplements may be essential in reducing the risks of deficiencies and supporting the foetus. Additionally, in some cases, menopausal women may also benefit from supplements in order to help manage some of the symptoms of the menopause.

In addition to special diets and our stage of life, deficiencies can also arise as a result of chronic stress and gastrointestinal dysfunction, which can negatively impact nutrient absorption and, of course, inadequate dietary intake.

As discussed in Chapter 9, stress is a major contributor to nutritional deficiencies in the modern world. During periods of chronic stress, the brain activates the sympathetic nervous system (SNS), which is responsible for our flight-or-fight mode. When the SNS is activated it reduces the activity of many biochemical processes that are required for everyday physiological function; for example, optimal digestion and reproductive capability are often lowered. Additionally, the SNS draws on our nutrient stores to synthesise a constant stream of the stress hormones cortisol, adrenaline and noradrenaline. Consequently, our nutritional demands drastically escalate and as a result this can pose a risk of nutritional deficiencies if those demands are not met. Our fight-or-flight mechanism is an imperative function for keeping us alive, but it was never intended to be activated for prolonged periods of time. As a result, we're often unable to provide the necessary nutrients required to sustain chronic periods of stress. Consequently, the resulting lack of nutrients can provide one explanation as to how chronic stress contributes to a suppressed immune system, poor sleep, impaired gut health and an increased risk of skin breakouts. In some individuals stress can suppress appetite, which causes an even greater risk of nutrient deficiencies.

Are Supplements a Good Safety Net?

Relying on supplements as a back-up support to the diet has become a common phenomenon. This is where individuals take a wide array of supplements as a precautionary measure, irrespective of dietary intake and often based on the common misconception that taking supplements will help to support general health and keep the lurgy away. Unfortunately, it's not quite that straightforward and if it were we would all experience far less illness. As we've just explored, taking supplements can come with its own challenges. The research around supplementation is diverse and the implications for us really depend on who we are and our nutritional status to begin with.

Should I be taking vitamin C?

Typically when we think of supplements and the immune system, vitamin C is the first one that comes to mind. However, are we placing too much emphasis on vitamin C supplements to support immunity? Can these supplements protect healthy individuals? Evidence has shown that taking a vitamin C supplement may help to reduce the risk of pneumonia and other serious respiratory infections in those are who deficient. Vitamin C supplementation has also been associated with a reduction in the severity of some diseases and death in individuals with low plasma vitamin C status.

Furthermore, high levels of stress increase the demand for vitamin C. As a result, those suffering with high stress may be at a greater risk of deficiency. There is some evidence that shows that taking a vitamin C supplement at the onset of a common cold significantly reduced the intensity of the symptoms in chronically stressed individuals. Similar research also shows that vitamin C supplementation can reduce the intensity and duration of symptoms. However, supplementing all year round may not provide you with any extra protection if you're already getting enough vitamin C through your diet. All this goes to show that you are far better off focusing on consuming your five portions of fruits and vegetables per day, as these are the most abundant sources of vitamin C and can ensure adequate intakes.

Should I be taking a vitamin D supplement?

As we discussed in Chapter 5, vitamin D plays a key role in the immune system, supporting the transportation of T-cells, the production of natural killer cells and the activation of T-reg cells.

Vitamin D deficiency is hugely prevalent in the UK due to the lack of sunshine (which is our primary source) throughout the winter months and the limited dietary sources of vitamin D. It is predominantly synthesised through exposure to UV rays from the sun so it stands to reason that vitamin D status is at its lowest at the end of the winter months and highest throughout the summer period.

Vitamin D took the world by storm during the Covid-19 pandemic as multiple research studies suggested that vitamin D reduced the rates of infection and improved outcomes from the infection. Although the factors influencing the individual outcomes of Covid-19 are far more complex than the individual's vitamin D status, it's undisputed that ensuring adequate vitamin D status is imperative for supporting a healthy immune system.

Evidence suggests that vitamin D deficiency has been associated with an increased risk of cardiovascular disease and autoimmune conditions such as type 1 diabetes and inflammatory bowel disease. Further research has also highlighted an association between low levels of vitamin D and an increased risk of respiratory infections in children.

In addition, vitamin D supplementation may be particularly crucial during pregnancy, as this is a peak period for programming the foetus's innate immune system. Evidence suggests that a higher dose of vitamin D during the second and third trimesters contributed to increased protection against infectious diseases and asthma during the early years. Most pregnancy multivitamins should contain adequate amounts of vitamin D; however, if you're concerned, seek personalised advice from your midwife.

Elderly individuals are at a greater risk of vitamin D deficiency as the ability to synthesise vitamin D from sunlight exposure declines with age. Additionally, the conversion of inactive vitamin D to active vitamin D is also weakened with age, which in turn has a negative impact on vitamin D status. Furthermore, elderly individuals may also be less likely to expose themselves to sunlight during the summer months.

The UK recommendation is to supplement with 10µg of vitamin D per day throughout the winter months between October and March. However, due to the instability of the weather in the UK, if the months outside of this are particularly dark and dreary then do consider supplementing during this period too.

Furthermore, there are many professionals who would argue that 10μg per day is not enough. However, high doses can pose a risk of toxicity.

Vitamin D supplements are generally found in two main forms: vitamin D2 (ergocalciferol) and vitamin D3 (cholecalciferol). Vitamin D3 has been consistently shown to be far more bioavailable and can often be found in two main sources: lichen and lanolin. Lichen is the plant-based vegan option which is derived from algae and lanolin is derived from sheep's wool. Since vitamin D is a fat-soluble nutrient, vitamin D supplements are best consumed with a meal containing healthy fats.

As with all supplements, if you're on medications or have underlying health conditions always seek advice from your GP.

What's the deal with magnesium?

Magnesium is one of the most abundant micronutrients in the human body and is required as a co-factor in over 700 physiological reactions. Magnesium is particularly important in supporting immune health and deficiency can significantly impact immune cell function. As magnesium plays a vital role in protecting against oxidative stress, deficiency can cause dysfunction of the endothelial cells in response to higher levels of oxidative stress and an increase in proinflammatory cytokines.

Despite the plethora of available dietary sources that contain magnesium, deficiency in the western world is still astonishingly common. Common magnesium-rich foods include green leafy vegetables, dark chocolate, nuts and seeds, avocados, beans and pulses.

Magnesium deficiency can occur due to a variety of circumstances, including in those who struggle with regular diarrhoea, a commonplace symptom for those who suffer with IBS-D (irritable bowel syndrome-diarrhoea). Magnesium deficiency can also be caused by low nutrient absorption due to an impaired gastrointestinal function, a diet high in ultra-processed foods and low in whole foods, and chronic stress. Deficiency can be identified through a blood test and common symptoms can include reduced appetite, impaired sleep, nausea and vomiting, weakness, fatigue and muscle cramps.

A magnesium deficiency shouldn't be a major cause for concern as it can be easily corrected. Evidence suggests that a suppressed immune function caused by magnesium deficiency can be reversed when supplementation is used to restore adequate magnesium status. Furthermore, magnesium deficiency is not uncommon in those with non-communicable diseases such as cardiovascular disease, diabetes, asthma, irritable bowel syndrome and neurodegenerative diseases, all of which can contribute to low-grade chronic inflammation. This parallel is important, as the evidence is not yet clear as to whether the non-communicable diseases increase magnesium utilisation (and consequently increase the risk of deficiency) or whether deficiency increases the risk of these diseases. What is clear is that magnesium deficiency can contribute to a damaged immune system and an increase in inflammation. Therefore, in cases where magnesium status is low or deficient, supplementation may be beneficial in supporting immune health.

Some magnesium supplements can contribute to gastrointestinal discomfort and consequently seeking personalised advice from your healthcare provider is essential. Another excellent way to top up your magnesium status is to add Epsom salts to your bath as the magnesium in the salts can be absorbed through the skin. It's recommended to soak in around ½–1 cup of Epsom salts in order to gain the benefits. However, Epsom salt baths alone are unlikely to reverse a deficiency.

Should I stock up on zinc?

Zinc has long been understood to play a vital role in immunomodulation. It's a key player in supporting the production of enzymes and their activities, cell proliferation and protein synthesis, including collagen production, all of which are essential in optimal wound healing. Additionally, zinc is required to support DNA replication and repair and is crucial to supporting healthy ageing. The elderly population are among those at the greatest risk of deficiency due to lower absorption rates and reduced dietary intakes.

Acute zinc deficiency has been associated with an increased risk of susceptibility to infection due to a suppression in the activity of the innate and adaptive immune cells. Furthermore, a chronic zinc deficiency contributes to an increase in pro-inflammatory cytokines and consequently a greater risk of chronic inflammatory diseases.

The correction of acute zinc deficiency through supplementation can help to restore the innate and adaptive immune cells back to their routine functioning. However, supplementation in cases where zinc status is sufficient can increase the risk of zinc toxicity. This backs up the notion that the role of supplementation is to correct deficiency rather than protect against contracting disease in those who are already consuming enough zinc in their diet.

Whenever you're considering supplementation it's always recommended that you seek advice from your healthcare professional as the type of supplement and timing of intake can be critical in the success of the supplement. If you are concerned about any aspect of your micronutrient status always seek advice from your GP. Most micronutrients can be assessed via a simple blood test and in many cases can be corrected accordingly.

Should I be taking a probiotic supplement to support my immune system?

Probiotics are types of live bacteria which can positively influence the host bacteria. Probiotics have taken the nation by storm and they're often deemed to be one of those super-supplements many believe will have the magic desired effect of 'fixing the gut'. While they can be beneficial for some individuals and for certain conditions and systems, they are not necessarily the magic answer.

Under the guidance of a healthcare professional, probiotics may be administered to help manage conditions such as gastro-intestinal disorders, irritable bowel syndrome, mental wellbeing, allergic diseases, atopic diseases and chronic diseases such as diabetes. For many of these conditions the initial evidence is promising, although far more research is needed into the mechanisms behind the effects of probiotics.

Furthermore, there are promising research papers which propose immunological benefits in response to probiotics. These benefits vary greatly depending on the targeted site of immunity and the genus, species and strain of the bacteria. The genus refers to the 'family' of bacteria and species and strain being the subcategories within the genus. The most commonly researched genera are *Lactobacillus*, *Bifidobacterium* and *Saccharomyces*, which are also some of the ones most often found in probiotic supplements.

Some types of probiotics have been found to directly interact with the immune cells and promote the production of cytokines. Additionally, some can help with stimulating the activity of the T-cells, which are involved in the secretion of the anti-inflammatory cytokine interleukin-10. Another proposed mechanism of action is that of increasing the production of the proteins which are required to maintain the integrity of the tight junctions in the gut lining. Consequently, this can promote a stronger gut barrier function. Furthermore, probiotics have been associated with amplifying the activity of the innate immune cells and modulating inflammation caused by unwanted pathogens.

Probiotics can also indirectly support immune cell function thorough increasing the growth and development of the commensal bacteria (good bacteria) and reducing the growth of the pathogenic bacteria (bad bacteria). This occurs as the beneficial live cultures compete for nutrients that would otherwise be utilised by the pathogenic species.

While the research into probiotics and immune function is particularly encouraging, it's still very much in its infancy and further research is required to understand which genera, strains and species are the most effective at modulating the immune system. Furthermore, our baseline microbiome may impact how we respond to probiotics on an individual level. It's important to highlight, therefore, that in some cases consuming probiotics can contribute to escalating undesirable symptoms. This is particularly the case if an individual consumes the wrong type of probiotics when they have small intestinal bacterial overgrowth (SIBO). This is a condition where bacteria grows in the small intestine and the wrong probiotics can contribute to feeding this unwanted overgrowth.

It's clear then that ensuring an appropriate high-quality probiotic is far more complicated than blindly grabbing one off a shelf. It can be a minefield as there are thousands of products containing a wide variety of bacteria, combinations of bacteria and dosages. In addition, in order to be effective, probiotics are required to survive the intense conditions of the gastrointestinal tract, such as the stomach acid and exposure to bile, before arriving in the gut microbiome. Once the bacteria arrive in the gut they must be able to colonise in order to survive and promote optimal wellbeing. The reality is that many probiotics on the market today are unable to arrive in the gut intact or may not be able to completely colonise it.

If you are interested in supplementing with probiotics, do seek advice from a healthcare professional to ensure you're obtaining the right probiotics. In the meantime, focus on consuming probiotic-rich foods and nourishing your gut through your diet and lifestyle habits.

Are protein supplements necessary for immunity?

The protein supplement industry is a multibillion-dollar industry and protein has now taken centre stage. We're often told that we're not consuming enough protein when the reality is that most of us are consuming adequate amounts. However, those who engage in intense training regimes, the elderly or individuals on a vegan or vegetarian diet may be at risk of protein deficiency.

Consequently, if you're concerned about your protein intake or you fall into any of the categories outlined above then supplementing with protein supplements can help to support your requirements. The important thing to remember when using protein supplements is that they should be used to supplement whole food dietary sources rather than replace them. Protein supplements are most commonly found in the form of drinks, powders or bars.

Furthermore, there are definitely differences in the health and nutrition aspects of the protein supplements on the market.

Many of the products commercially available to us (particularly the more mainstream brands that we regularly see on supermarket shelves) are laden with food additives, sweeteners, fillers and bulking agents. As we explored in Chapter 7, an overconsumption of food additives, artificial ingredients and artificial sweeteners can contribute to inflammatory responses and modulation of immune cell activity. Furthermore, many of these products contain sugar alcohols to provide sweetness and bulk. Sugar alcohols are well known to disrupt gastrointestinal function, particularly in those with gastrointestinal disorders and irritable bowel syndrome.

Therefore, if you are looking to support your diet with some protein supplements, try to opt for those which contain no artificial additives or bulking agents and are free from artificial sweeteners. Unflavoured protein powders are your best options to meet these requirements. Be aware that the source of protein in these products varies greatly. The most common sources of protein used in protein supplements include whey, casein, soya, rice, pea and hemp. Tolerance for each source can vary between individuals so ensure you find the right protein source for you.

While it's clear that there can be a role for dietary supplements, it's important to remember that they should be used to *supplement* rather than *replace* whole foods. Hopefully this chapter has highlighted some of the key factors to think about. The dose, type, nutrient composition and your individual medical situation should all be taken into account when choosing supplements. In most cases, we can all benefit from taking the recommended 10µg of vitamin D per day throughout the winter months. Additionally, those following a vegetarian or vegan diet may also benefit from supplementing with higher-risk nutrients. Generally, individuals suffering with high levels of stress, pregnant women and those with certain conditions or deficiencies may also benefit.

There may also be situations where certain nutrients can support the immune system; however, we needn't all be taking a concoction of supplements every morning. Do remember that taking any dietary supplement should always be approached with caution. If you're on medication, the contraceptive pill or have a medical condition, it's vital you speak to your healthcare provider to ensure there are no risks of drug–nutrient interaction or other possible side effects.

Summary Points

- A 'food first' approach is always preferable since foods contain many other benefits alongside the nutrient of interest. Nutrients in foods are often found within a matrix of co-factors, which can help aid absorption.
- The overconsumption of supplements can increase the risk of toxicity, impair absorption of other critical nutrients, contribute to adverse health effects and increase the stress placed on the liver.
- Supplements come in a variety of forms, some of which can contribute to undesirable side effects such as changes in bowel movements and nausea.
- In some cases, supplements can be hugely beneficial for reducing the risk of or reversing a deficiency. This is where supplements may play a role in supporting immune function.

- There is some promising evidence to support the use of probiotics for immunity; however, the specific types of bacteria required are not fully understood yet.
- In the UK it's recommended to supplement 10µg of vitamin D per day between October and March.
- Protein supplements can be used to support protein intake but it's not advisable to replace whole food protein sources with protein bars or powders.

CHAPTER 11

Practical Ways to Support Your Immunity

In this chapter, I'll focus on tying all the information in the book together to provide you with the tools to support your immune system when it has come under attack and bring it back to recovery. Despite the fact there is no quick fix for preventing or recovering from illness, our diet and lifestyle behaviours can definitely positively or negatively influence our ability to deal with illness and any associated symptoms during these times.

You can use the information in this chapter as your go-to quick guide when you're feeling low or are struggling with an illness. Feel free to tear out the pages and stick them on your fridge or wherever feels most useful. Sometimes thinking about incorporating advice into your diet and lifestyle when you're feeling less than your normal self can be challenging. This is why I've done the work for you. Here are the practical tips that encompass all of the science I've highlighted throughout the book. I really hope they can be of great help in times of need.

Remember, though, don't put too much pressure on yourself

when you're feeling low. Allow yourself time to nourish your body in order to optimise your recovery.

I've also included some of my recipes to encourage and inspire you to nourish your body and soul in an enjoyable way. I'm no cordon bleu chef but I am an enthusiastic home cook and for this reason you won't find recipes that are overly complicated, that require you to spend hours in the kitchen or to have weird and wacky ingredients or appliances. They're here to show you how eating nutritious food really can be quick, delicious and exciting. They are all highly adaptable so you can alter them according to the ingredients you have available to you.

Five Things You Can Do When You Feel Your Immune System Is Under Attack

We're all familiar with the feeling of being run-down and the sense that we're about to fall victim to an attacking pathogen. This situation often occurs as a result of running ourselves into the ground or spreading our efforts so thinly that we've forgotten to take care of ourselves.

As discussed, it's not about 'boosting' our immune system to protect us in times like these and unfortunately there's no magic cure or pill we can take to prevent getting ill. However, there are some habits which you can adopt to support your immune system to function optimally and fight off unwanted pathogens.

1. Hydrate

Hydration is vital for assisting the immune system in carrying out the necessary tasks. If you're dehydrated you're less likely to be able to transport key nutrients around the body that are required for their numerous roles within the immune cells. Additionally, hydration is an important component in helping to excrete unwanted pathogens.

Vomiting and diarrhoea are common symptoms of illness and can contribute to a significant risk of dehydration due to increased fluid losses. As a result, ensuring you're staying hydrated when your immune system is feeling compromised is vital. The recommendations are to consume around 2 litres of water per day, although during very hot weather or if you're particularly active you may require slightly more. As a reminder, overhydration can also be detrimental to your health, so make sure you're drinking to satisfy your thirst rather than aiming for an excessive water intake. Consuming too much fluid can disrupt the electrolyte balance in the body and may contribute to some adverse side effects.

2. Prioritise sleep

As discussed in Chapter 9, sleep is paramount to supporting your immune system. Sleep deprivation can often be a contributing factor to weakening the immune system and increasing susceptibility to an attack from unwanted pathogens.

Sleep is a critical period for your body to reset and regenerate the immune cells. Consequently, ensuring you have ample amounts of sleep is essential, particularly when you're running on empty. In some cases, you may need to cut back on your daily tasks, skip a workout or cancel a social arrangement to fit in a few extra hours of sleep. That's more than OK. In fact, it's a non-negotiable when it comes to supporting your immune system and your general health and wellbeing.

3. Eat your five a day

You know by now that fruits and vegetables are rich sources of fibre, phytochemicals and key nutrients, all of which are required to support your immune system. They're one of the most abundant sources of vitamin C, which can help to reduce the duration and severity of symptoms of the common cold or flu. Snacking on fruit and vegetables or opting for a vegetable-packed soup can be a really simple, easy and accessible way to increase your vitamin C intake when you're feeling run-down.

4. Increase prebiotic- and probiotic-rich foods

Despite what the food and supplement industry tells us, probiotics are far from a magic fix. However, as we have explored throughout these pages, the gut plays a central role in supporting immune health. Therefore, nourishing the gut with prebiotic- and probiotic-rich foods can be an excellent way to support your gut during a period of heightened stress. Adding garlic, leeks and onions to your recipes and incorporating live yoghurt, kefir and kombucha into your daily routine are all excellent ways to show your gut that extra bit of love throughout this time.

5. Reduce your sugar intake

Often when feeling run-down we experience fatigue and a lack of energy. It's in these situations that we see an increase in sugar cravings. Be aware that fuelling your body with sugar at this time can contribute to blood sugar spikes and crashes which over time may contribute to increased inflammation. As a result, it's imperative to try to limit our sugar intake at these times.

If this is something which feels challenging for you, go back to Chapter 7, where I discuss blood sugar balancing, as the information there can help you to reduce the blood glucose spikes and crashes.

Remember, these tips are not a magic bullet so don't expect to be invincible if you're consistently neglecting your health and wellbeing to the point where it's challenged. This advice will definitely help you up to a point but do remember that it's the dietary and lifestyle behaviours which you engage in on a daily basis that will support you the most. Throughout the book there are so many tips and tricks for optimising your immunity and your wellbeing. By incorporating these into your day-to-day behaviours you're much more likely to benefit overall than if you simply lean into these quick tips when you're feeling low.

Five Ways to Support Your Recovery After an Acute Illness

By this point you're hopefully on the other side of an acute illness. Your immune system has been under fire and you've been working hard to fight off unwanted pathogens. However, in the process you're likely to have felt run-down, tired and far from the best version of yourself. As a result, as soon as you start feeling like yourself again you'll want to get back to day-to-day normality (although sometimes bouncing back too quickly can be detrimental to ongoing improvement). Here are my tips for ensuring you can support your recovery as smoothly and as optimally as possible.

1. Walk, don't run

Rushing back into a busy lifestyle when you're still warding off a cold or flu can cause you to take a few steps backwards. A busy lifestyle can contribute to increased levels of stress, which uses up more nutrients and therefore leaves fewer reserves for the immune system. Where possible, try to keep stress levels relatively low and avoid overcommitting. Ensure you're still leaving extra time to support your sleep needs to allow you to nurture a full recovery.

2. Renourish your body

If you've been ill, it's not uncommon to experience a reduced appetite which can leave you feeling slightly undernourished. A suppressed appetite during acute illness often occurs as a result of an increase in the proinflammatory cytokine, interleukin-8 (IL-8). Where possible, opt for plain but nutritious foods to support your requirements and to help navigate any nutrient shortfalls. A few simple meal ideas include:

- Vegetable-packed omelettes (try to include greens such as spinach, kale or spring greens).
- A bowl of porridge or overnight oats topped with banana and cinnamon.
- Sourdough toast with avocado or peanut butter.
- A berry-packed smoothie with nut butter, ground flax-seeds, yoghurt and some greens too!
- A nourishing bowl of vegetable soup.

3. Move your body

Overexercising when you're unwell is not recommended as exercise increases stress on the body and utilises more nutrients which could otherwise be used for the repair and recovery process. Taking the opportunity to rest when you're ill is far more effective. However, when you start to feel better, going outside for a walk, engaging in a gentle yoga or Pilates class or going for a light jog (if you're feeling up to it) are all great ways to release endorphins and to help support your immune system on its way to recovery.

4. Avoid alcohol

The metabolism of alcohol requires excess nutrients and can therefore draw on the very valuable stores needed to support your recovery. Drinking alcohol can also disrupt your sleep quality and quantity which can further impair recovery. Moreover, alcohol can also disturb your bowel movements which might just be returning to normal following an acute illness. Switch your alcoholic drinks for sparkling water and fresh lime, a refreshing and gut-nourishing kombucha or a cup of herbal tea. Have a look at the recipes in this book for some delicious alternatives to alcoholic drinks.

5. Practise your hygiene

I'd like to hope we're all practising hygiene on a daily basis, but recovering from an illness is an even more pertinent time to be washing your hands regularly. In times of recovery you want to allow your immune cells to focus on recovering and generating antibodies. Throwing more pathogens into the mix can generate more work for the immune cells which can make it harder for them to focus on the priority.

When your body is next trying to recover from a cold or flu illness, remember to use these tips. While they're far from a magic cure, they will remind you of some of the healthier habits which can support the body's repair and recovery. This can also be a great time to reinstate any habits that may have fallen by the wayside throughout the period of illness.

IMMUNE-FRIENDLY RECIPES

Breakfast

Shakshuka

This is one of my all-time favourite breakfasts and it's rich in a wide variety of polyphenols, prebiotic fibres, proteins and micronutrients. These ingredients are the perfect concoction for supporting your immune health. The onions and garlic are great sources of prebiotics and the array of spices provides a wide range of plant chemicals to support diet diversity, both of which can contribute to nourishing the gut bacteria. The eggs are also rich in a wide range of immune supporting nutrients such as protein, vitamin D, selenium and zinc.

Serves 2
1 tbsp olive oil
1 garlic clove, crushed

1 white onion, sliced

1 red pepper, sliced

1 courgette, sliced

1 portobello mushroom, sliced

3 tsp paprika

1 tsp smoked paprika

3 tsp ground cumin

1 tsp chilli flakes

2 x 400g tins chopped tomatoes

4 eggs

Sea salt and black pepper

1. Heat the olive oil in a pan over a medium heat, then add the garlic and sauté for 1–2 minutes. Add the onion, red pepper, courgette and mushroom with all the spices and a generous pinch of salt and pepper. Continue to cook over a medium heat for 3–4 minutes.

2. Once the vegetables have softened slightly, add the chopped tomatoes and leave to simmer over a low heat for a further 5–10 minutes.

3. Next, create four wells in the tomato sauce and crack in the eggs. Place a lid over the pan and leave over a low-medium heat for 8–10 minutes (depending on how soft you like your eggs).

4. Serve with fresh sourdough bread and enjoy.

Top tip: If you don't eat eggs, you can sprinkle tofu or feta cheese over the top instead.

Breakfast Smoothie

This smoothie is ideal for a quick breakfast before work. If you're really short on time I recommend adding all the ingredients to your blender the night before and just whizzing it up in the morning. The berries provide a source of polyphenols and the nut butter is rich in healthy fats which can help to support the structure of the immune cell membranes. Additionally, flaxseeds are a source of plant-based omega-3 which can help with promoting the anti-inflammatory response.

Serves 1
400ml milk of your choice
100g frozen berries
1 tbsp almond or peanut butter
1 tbsp natural yoghurt
1 tbsp milled flaxseeds
1 medjool date
¼ tsp ground cinnamon

1. Add all the ingredients to a high-speed blender and whizz until smooth. Pour out into a glass and enjoy.

Top tip: You can try mixing up the milks and nut butters in order to increase diversity in the diet. When you're buying nut butter try to avoid those with added sugar, glucose syrup or palm oil.

Vanilla and Strawberry Overnight Oats

This is another quick, easy, nutritious and of course really delicious breakfast for those busier mornings. It's also one you can make in batches to feed the family or to see you through the week. Similarly to flaxseeds, chia seeds are a rich plant source of omega-3. Yoghurt and milk (if you're using dairy) provide nutrients such as calcium and iodine. Iodine is particularly important in promoting metabolism and managing the balance of proinflammatory and anti-inflammatory mediators. Oats are high in fibre and are a very good source of plant-based iron, which plays a role in managing the cells of the adaptive immune system. Furthermore, the vitamin C in the strawberries can help to increase the absorption of the iron from the oats.

Serves 1
50g jumbo oats
2 tbsp chia seeds
2 tbsp natural yoghurt
250ml milk of your choice
½ tsp vanilla extract
80g strawberries, diced

1. Add the oats and chia seeds to a bowl and combine well.
2. Stir through the yoghurt, milk and vanilla extract and combine well. You can add the strawberries to the mix now or save them to scatter on top when you serve.
3. Cover the bowl or place the mix into an airtight container and store in the fridge overnight. In the morning, your breakfast is ready to go!

Top tips: Serve this with some peanut butter for extra protein and healthy fats.

If you're making this in bulk, double or triple the recipe.

For a vegan option use a dairy-free milk and a yoghurt alternative.

Tahini Granola

Granola is a delicious way to incorporate a wide variety of plant foods into your diet. It also happens to be a quick and convenient option for breakfast when you're rushing out the door. Unfortunately, many shop-bought granolas can be very high in sugar. Making your own granola is far more cost-effective and you can moderate the amount of sugar to your liking. This recipe contains a variety of diverse ingredients and is rich in omega-3 to help support that vital omega-3 to omega-6 ratio. Nuts and seeds are excellent sources of fibre, protein and healthy fats, all of which contribute to supporting the immune system. Furthermore, fibre is particularly important for nourishing those gut microbes. Tahini also provides some calcium and plant-based iron.

Makes 10–12
250g oats
100g walnuts
60g almonds
25g linseeds
60g pumpkin seeds
100g raisins
Pinch of salt
½ tsp ground cinnamon

35g avocado oil
70g honey or maple syrup
125g tahini

1. Preheat the oven to 180°C/gas mark 4 and line a large baking tray with baking parchment.
2. Add all the dry ingredients in a bowl and stir to combine.
3. Pour the avocado oil, honey or maple syrup and tahini into another bowl and mix well.
4. Pour the wet ingredients into the dry ingredients and stir until all the dry ingredients are fully coated.
5. Pour the granola out on to the lined baking tray and bake in the oven for 20–25 minutes, stirring half-way through.
6. Once the granola is cooked, turn the oven off and leave to cool inside the oven (this helps the granola to crisp up).

Top tip: This recipe is really flexible and you can use whatever nuts and seeds you have in the cupboard. Jumbo oats are a better option than porridge oats as they release their carbs more slowly into the bloodstream. You can swap the tahini for any other nut or seed butter.

Veggie Baked Omelette

This veggie-filled omelette is a superb option for breakfast, brunch, lunch or even a light dinner. You can make it ahead of time, too, if you've got a busy day. Eggs are a rich source of protein, vitamin B12 and choline.

Peas are one of my favourite ingredients as they can be kept in the freezer and so are always to hand. They're rich in plant-based protein and contain vitamin K and zinc. You can also play around with adding any other vegetables and herbs you may have as this can help to promote diversity.

Serves 3–4
1 large sweet potato, diced
1 white onion, thinly sliced
1 tsp avocado oil
8 eggs
100g peas (if frozen, cover with boiling water and then drain before using)
1 tbsp mixed herbs
Sea salt and black pepper

1. Preheat the oven to 180°C/gas mark 4.
2. Arrange the diced sweet potato and sliced onion on a baking tray, drizzle over the avocado oil and season with a pinch of salt and pepper. Roast in the oven for 15–20 minutes.
3. Meanwhile, crack the eggs into a bowl and whisk well. Add the mixed herbs, peas and some seasoning and whisk again.
4. Once the roasted vegetables are soft, remove them from the oven and allow to cool slightly. Transfer them to a lined brownie tin and pour over the egg mix.
5. Bake the omelette in the oven for about 30 minutes. Leave to cool before slicing up and serving. Enjoy!

Top tip: This is lovely served with salad and sourdough toast. You can also add feta or grated Cheddar to the egg mix if you wanted to increase the protein and calcium content.

Smoky Beans on Sourdough with Garlic Mushrooms and Spinach

These smoky beans are a healthier version of the nation's favourite baked beans on toast. The beans and the garlic provide a rich source of prebiotic fibres to help nourish your gut while the spinach is rich in plant-based iron, vitamin C and vitamin K. You can of course mix up the beans you use in this recipe.

Real sourdough bread contains prebiotic fibres and live cultures and can be easier for some individuals to digest since many of the gluten proteins are already broken down through the fermentation process. Remember that sourdough does still contain gluten and therefore those with coeliac disease should avoid it.

Serves 2
2 tsp avocado oil
½ tsp ground cumin
½ tsp paprika
1 tsp smoked paprika
1 x 400g tin butter beans, drained and rinsed
2 garlic cloves, crushed
150g mushrooms, sliced
100g spinach
4 slices of sourdough bread
Sea salt and black pepper
Fresh coriander, to serve

1. Heat one teaspoon of the avocado oil in a pan and add the cumin, paprika, smoked paprika and a generous pinch of salt and pepper. Leave to cook for a minute or so over a medium heat.

2. Next, add the butter beans to the pan, stir well to coat them in the spices and oil and leave to cook over a low-medium heat for 4–5 minutes.

3. Meanwhile, heat the remaining teaspoon of oil in a frying pan and add the garlic. Stir for a minute or so, then add the mushrooms along with a pinch of salt and pepper.

4. Once the mushrooms are soft, add the spinach and leave for one minute to wilt while you toast your sourdough bread.

5. Spoon the mushrooms and spinach over the toast, then top with the beans and some fresh coriander. Enjoy!

Lunch and Dinner

Buckwheat Wraps

While this recipe can be made with any flour, buckwheat is naturally gluten free and is higher in protein than white flour. The wraps can be made the night before and taken to work the next day. If you exclude the herbs, salt and pepper, the wrap batter can be used as a base for pancakes if you fancy a sweeter option. Avocado is a great source of monounsaturated fats and vitamin E. Vitamin E is a potent antioxidant and can help to neutralise free radicals in the body, which can otherwise contribute to attacking healthy cells and cells of the immune system.

Serves 2
100g buckwheat flour
2 eggs
90ml milk of your choice
1 tsp dried basil
1 tsp dried coriander
1 tsp avocado oil
2 tbsp smoky hummus (see page 247)
1 avocado, peeled, stoned and sliced
80g spinach
80g cherry tomatoes, halved
80g cucumber, sliced
Handful of fresh basil or coriander
Sea salt and black pepper

1. In a bowl, whisk together the buckwheat flour with the eggs, milk, dried basil, dried coriander and some salt and pepper.
2. Heat the oil in a frying pan; once heated, add one ladle of the wrap mix to the pan and tilt the pan to spread it over the surface. Cook for 2–3 minutes over a low-medium heat. Once you start to see bubbles on the surface, flip the wrap over and cook for a further 1–2 minutes. Repeat this process until you've used up all the mix.
3. Spread the hummus over to the base of each wrap and then layer the vegetables and fresh herbs on to

one side of the wrap. Roll the wrap up, slice in half and enjoy!

Top tip: You could add chicken strips or falafel to this wrap to increase the protein or fibre content.

Brown Rice Spaghetti with Homemade Avocado Pesto

Many of us aren't short of wheat in our diet, so mixing up our carbohydrate and grain sources is an excellent way to incorporate different plant compounds and increase variety in your diet. This recipe is incredibly quick and fuss free and it's also a great one to share as a family. The avocado, olive oil and walnuts are rich in healthy fats to help support the structures of the immune cells, although you can easily make it without the walnuts if you're cooking for someone with a nut allergy.

Serves 3
225g dried brown rice spaghetti
1½ large avocados
30g fresh basil, plus a few leaves to serve
4 tbsp olive oil
Juice of ½ lemon
1 large garlic clove
Generous pinch of salt
50g walnuts
Grated Parmesan or Cheddar, to serve

1. Cook the pasta in a large pan of boiling salted water, following the instructions on the packet.

2. Meanwhile, put the avocado, fresh basil, olive oil, lemon juice and garlic clove into a blender and blitz until smooth. Then pulse in the walnuts until they're slightly broken down but still provide some crunch.

3. Drain the pasta, then return to the pan along with the pesto sauce. Heat over a low-medium heat for 2–3 minutes, stirring gently to coat the spaghetti in the sauce.

4. Serve topped with a few extra basil leaves and your cheese of choice.

Top tip: If you're making this for more people you can double or triple the pesto recipe. You can also try green pea pasta, red lentil pasta and buckwheat pasta too, to increase diversity in the diet.

Immune-friendly Shepherd's Pie

Shepherd's pie is a common family favourite and while it's typically a 'meat and potatoes' type of dish, it can also offer a fantastic opportunity for incorporating a wide range of plant ingredients, beans and vegetables. You can also use the base to serve with pasta, making this the perfect 'cook once and eat twice' recipe. Beans are an excellent, affordable, high-protein, high-fibre ingredient. They're rich in plant compounds and play an important role in feeding a healthy gut microbiome.

Serves 4
2 large sweet potatoes, peeled and cubed
1 swede, peeled and cubed
1 tbsp avocado oil
1 large white onion, thinly sliced
1 leek, thinly sliced

3 celery sticks, thinly sliced

4 large carrots, diced

1 tbsp dried rosemary

1 tbsp dried thyme

1 tsp dried tarragon

2 tbsp tomato purée

500g mince of your choice

1 x 400g tin green lentils

100g peas

Sea salt and black pepper

1. Preheat the oven to 180°C/gas mark 4.
2. Add the cubed sweet potato and swede to a steaming basket and steam for 10 minutes until soft.
3. Heat the avocado oil in a pan, then add the onion, leek, celery and carrots, along with the dried herbs and a pinch of salt and pepper. Cook over a medium heat for 4–5 minutes until the vegetables have softened slightly.
4. Add the tomato purée with the mince and stir well. Cook for a further 4–5 minutes, stirring regularly to prevent burning.
5. Meanwhile, drain the lentils, add them to the pan and stir well. Cover with a lid and leave over a low heat while you drain and mash the sweet potatoes and swede. Season with salt and pepper.
6. Stir the peas into the mince mixture and then pour the mix into an ovenproof dish before evenly spreading the vegetable mash on top. Draw lines in the mash with a fork to allow for a crispy topping. Bake in the oven for

20–25 minutes, or until the mash goes slightly golden on top. Serve and enjoy.

Top tip: For a vegan option, omit the mince and add a tin of butter beans or extra lentils. If you are using mince, try mixing up between beef and lamb and pork, or use chicken or turkey for a leaner option.

Chicken Drumstick Tray Bake

This recipe is one for the family when you've walked in from work late. It's very quick, delicious and incorporates a wide range of spices to help support your immune system. You can always mix up the meat you're using or try it with chicken breasts and thighs, although you may need to adjust the cooking time. Chicken is a great source of vitamin B12. Avoiding vitamin B12 deficiency is imperative for promoting a healthy immune system.

Serves 4
8 chicken drumsticks
2 large red onions, cut into sixths
2 large sweet potatoes, sliced into wedges
2 aubergines, sliced into wedges
4 parsnips, sliced into wedges
2 tbsp avocado oil
1 x 400g tin chopped tomatoes
2 tsp ground cumin
1 tsp ground coriander
½ tsp ground cinnamon
1 tsp ground turmeric
Sea salt and black pepper

1. Preheat the oven to 180°C/gas mark 4.
2. Arrange the chicken drumsticks and all the vegetables on a large baking tray.
3. Put the avocado oil, chopped tomatoes, spices and some salt and pepper in a bowl and stir well. Then pour this mix over the vegetables and the chicken drumsticks and bake in the oven for 40 minutes.
4. Serve this on its own or with rice or quinoa. Enjoy!

Top tip: Try to cut the vegetables fairly large, to prevent burning and to ensure they all cook evenly. Note the vegetables will naturally shrink slightly.

Drinks and Soups

Matcha Latte

Matcha is a pure green tea powder which reaps a wide range of benefits to support the immune system. Most notably, matcha is high in polyphenols and antioxidants, which can help to protect against free radicals and high levels of oxidative stress.

While matcha does contain caffeine, it is present in lower amounts than in coffee beans. Additionally, the caffeine in matcha is released far more slowly into the bloodstream so, rather than experiencing a sharp rise and fall in energy, as you would with coffee, you're more likely to see a gradual rise followed by a gentle decline.

Serves 1

1 tsp matcha powder

2 tbsp cold water

250ml milk of your choice

1. Begin by adding the matcha powder to a mug.
2. Next add the cold water and using a matcha whisk (or regular whisk), very gently whisk the powder into the water until you have a very smooth paste.
3. Heat the milk in a pan or in a milk jug; once it's heated through, add the milk to the mug and enjoy.

Top tip: Try to buy a pure, high-quality matcha powder where you can. Some lower-quality matcha powders contain sugars and are lower in plant chemicals and antioxidants.

You can also make this into a tea by switching the milk for water, although avoid boiling the milk or the water as this can scald the matcha and degrade its beneficial properties.

You can also make this iced by using cold water or milk and adding ice to the glass.

Rosemary Spritz

Reducing your alcohol consumption is a fantastic step to supporting your immune health, although this is definitely something that is easier said than done. However, having delicious alternative drinks is a great way to help to encourage you to make those healthier choices. If you're looking for something delicious, hydrating and refreshing then look no further.

Serves 1
½ tsp rose water
Juice of ½ lime
250ml sparkling water
1–2 sprigs of fresh rosemary
2–3 ice cubes
Lime wedge, to garnish

1. Add the rose water and lime juice to a glass and stir gently. Top up with the sparkling water and finish off with the fresh rosemary and ice cubes.
2. Make a small cut into the flesh of the lime wedge and place on the side of the glass. Add a straw and enjoy.

Top tip: Serving this in a gin glass or a long glass can make it feel that bit more special and exciting.

Refreshing Green Juice

This juice is the perfect way to stay hydrated and refreshed on the days where you're looking for something that bit more enticing. It's rich in plant compounds and high-water-content fruits and vegetables which can really help to support your hydration requirements.

Serves 1–2
2 green apples
½ cucumber
1 celery stick
Juice of ½ lime

1. Add all the ingredients to a juicer and serve in a glass with a few ice cubes.

Top tip: If your palate can tolerate a slightly less sweet flavour, you can switch the apples for courgette.

Nourishing Greens Soup

The courgettes, broccoli and spinach are all packed full of vitamin C and plant-based iron. The range of herbs can also contribute to diversifying your dietary intake, and it's ideal for making in batches and storing in the freezer for a rainy day.

Serves 3–4
1 tbsp avocado oil
1 large white onion, thinly sliced
3 celery sticks, thinly sliced
1 tbsp dried rosemary
2 tsp dried basil
2 tsp dried thyme
2 courgettes, chopped
1 head of broccoli, chopped
1 litre vegetable stock
200g spinach
Juice of ½ lemon
Sea salt and black pepper

1. Heat the avocado oil in a pan over a medium heat.
2. Add the onion and celery to the pan along with the

rosemary, basil and thyme. Sauté for a few minutes until the onion turns translucent.

3. Add the courgettes and broccoli to the pan along with the stock and season with salt and pepper. Cover with a lid and leave to simmer over a low-medium heat for 10–15 minutes.

4. Add the spinach and continue to heat for 1–2 minutes to soften down, then transfer the soup to a high-speed blender with the lemon juice and whizz until smooth (be careful here as it can splatter; depending on the size of your blender you may need to do this in two batches).

5. Serve and enjoy.

Top tip: This soup is delicious served with a spoon of natural yoghurt or topped with roasted chickpeas for a source of protein and an extra crunch.

Creamy Roasted Tomato Soup

This creamy roasted tomato soup is a healthier take on a British favourite. It's rich in the plant compound lycopene which provides the vibrant red colour to the tomatoes. Lycopene has powerful antioxidant capabilities to help support a healthier immune system. This recipe is pretty hands-off so is perfect if you're looking to catch up on some admin at the same time.

Serves 3–4
1kg tomatoes, quartered
2 large white onions, quartered
3 garlic cloves

1 tbsp avocado oil

2 tbsp mixed herbs

300ml hot vegetable stock

Sea salt and black pepper

1. Preheat the oven to 180°C/gas mark 4.
2. Place the tomatoes and onions on a baking tray with the peeled garlic cloves. Coat well with the avocado oil and mixed herbs and season with salt and pepper.
3. Roast in the oven for 35–40 minutes until the onions and tomatoes are soft and juicy.
4. Add the contents of the baking tray (including any liquid) to a blender along with the stock and whizz until smooth. Season with salt and pepper to taste and enjoy.

Snacks

Fig and Walnut Energy Balls

These energy balls can be made ahead of time and stored in an airtight container to be enjoyed throughout the week. The walnuts are a good source of omega-3 and protein while the figs are rich in fibre and plant-based iron. The protein in the walnuts can also help to slow down the release of sugars into the bloodstream.

Makes 8–10
100g walnuts
50g almonds
200g dried figs
Pinch of salt
50g desiccated coconut, for rolling

1. Add the walnuts and almonds to a food processor and blitz until they're slightly crushed.
2. Add the dried figs and the salt to the mix and blend until a dough-like texture occurs.
3. Roll into balls and then coat them in the desiccated coconut. Place in the fridge for 2–3 hours then enjoy.

Top tip: For the best results use partially rehydrated figs. You can switch up the nuts and dried fruit you use in this recipe to use whatever you have in the cupboard and to diversify your diet. Dried dates or dried apricots work really well instead of the figs.

Chocolatey Oatcakes

These chocolatey oatcakes can be an ideal, fibre-rich way to enjoy a sweet boost of energy in the afternoons. They're also delicious as an after-dinner dessert. Where possible try to use as high of a percentage of dark chocolate as you can as the darker the chocolate, the less sugar and higher cocoa concentration there is. Cocoa (in its purest form) is rich in polyphenols and plant chemicals, which can have antioxidant effects to help support the immune system. Additionally, the peanut butter and hemp seeds provide healthy fats and contain protein.

Serves 2
50g dark chocolate
1 banana
4 oatcakes
1 tbsp peanut butter
1 tbsp hemp seeds

1. Melt the dark chocolate in a heatproof bowl, over a bowl of just simmering water.
2. Slice the banana into coins.
3. Spread the peanut butter on the oatcakes and top with hemp seeds and banana slices. Finish off by drizzling the dark chocolate over the oatcakes. Place in the fridge for 30 minutes to set.

Top tip: You can use another nut or seed butter instead of peanut butter. Also try mixing up the hemp seeds with flaxseeds or sesame seeds. These are also delicious with sliced strawberries instead of banana.

Smoky Hummus

Not only is hummus a delicious addition to roasted vegetables, it's also a perfect appetiser and all-round staple in my diet. It's also a high-protein, high-fibre dish which can be hugely versatile as you can add a wide array of flavours and vegetables to the mix in order to promote diversity and keep your diet interesting. This is a simple recipe for a smoky hummus, although you can always add roasted sweet potatoes or butternut squash to increase its bulk, fibre and micronutrient profile.

Chickpeas are another great source of prebiotics, which help to nourish the beneficial bacteria in the gut.

Serves 4
1x 400g tin chickpeas
1 garlic clove
Juice of 2 lemons
3 heaped tbsp tahini paste
1 tbsp water
2 tbsp olive oil
1 tsp smoked paprika
Sea salt, to taste

1. Drain the chickpeas, then add to a blender or food processor with all the remaining ingredients. Blend until smooth.
2. Store in an airtight container in the fridge.

Top tip: This will store in the fridge for a few days and can be enjoyed as a snack with vegetable crudités, oatcakes or rice cakes. It's also great added to salads, sandwiches, wraps and roasted vegetables, for an extra hit of protein.

Five Things to Take Away From This Book

Whether you've read this book from cover to cover or you've used it as a guide to flick through to the subjects which interest you the most, there are a few final comments and essential principles which I would love to leave you with. If you take nothing else away from this book, these five key points are essential to bear in mind when you're thinking about your immune system. Feel free to tear this page out and stick it in a place where you'll constantly be reminded.

1. There are no magic cures or quick fixes

I'm sure by now you've got this message as I really have hammered this home and I don't apologise for my repetition of this. All too often the basics aren't prioritised and far too much time or money is spent on putting a plaster over the effects caused by our current dietary and lifestyle behaviours. To put it succinctly: a magic cure or a quick fix quite simply doesn't exist.

2. Your gut health plays a key role in your overall health and immune system

Despite all the product claims and probiotics on the market, focusing on your habits and daily diet is the best place to start when it comes to supporting your gut health. Of course, probiotics and gut support supplements can play a role when they've been advised by a professional but if you're not starting with basic good habits, there's nothing you can take that will overhaul your gut health in the long term.

3. Plants are ESSENTIAL to supporting a healthy immune system

We shouldn't underestimate the benefits of eating plants on health and our immunity. Plants are a powerful way to incorporate diversity into our diet. They're rich in a wide range of micronutrients and polyphenols and they're also excellent for increasing our fibre consumption. Try to broaden your horizons by incorporating one new plant food per week or month into your diet. Not only will this help to improve your wellbeing and the health of your immune system, it can also help to expand your palette.

4. Don't underestimate the power of sleep!

Sleep really can be your best friend when it comes to optimising your immune system. As a reminder, it has been deemed to be more important to our long-term overall health than diet and exercise combined. It's easy for us to scrimp on sleep when we have a multitude of tasks to do. However, we can all sense when we're feeling run-down as a result of sleep deprivation. If you know you're not getting enough sleep, try to add an extra hour to the time spent in bed. This can be as simple as going to bed thirty minutes earlier and waking up thirty minutes later. Not only will your immune system thank you in the long run but you may also find that your energy increases and as a result your everyday functioning improves too. You will also be a whole lot better equipped to help ward off disease and infection.

5. Pick one habit you want to change

Many of us have habits which we'd like to change. Whether it's making an extra effort to reduce your cigarette smoking or alcohol consumption, prioritising an extra 15 minutes of walking each day or reducing your consumption of sugar or artificially sweetened beverages, there really are changes that everyone can make. What's more, these needn't cost you a whole lot of time or money to implement.

In recent years there has been an explosion of knowledge and interest in the area of nutrition science. We're only at the beginning of understanding such a complex subject area, but these points can help set your health and wellbeing on the right trajectory. I have no doubt that we have so much more to learn to build on the knowledge we already have. Although, it's definitely an exciting time for this area of research.

Conclusion

We're extremely fortunate to live in a world which offers us such a wide range of joyful activities and luxuries, although it's now clear that our modern world is simultaneously a major driving factor in the increased incidences of metabolic syndrome and autoimmune conditions. It's also an important explanation for the increase in our susceptibility to common illnesses and diseases. As long as the modern world continues to advance and develop in the way that it has done thus far, some of the adverse influences on our immune system will remain outside of our control. On the plus side, as we've explored in this book, there are so many factors and habits which remain within our control.

We currently have much more information and understanding about the relationship between the gut and the immune system, although I have no doubt that this area of research is constantly evolving and we're sure to learn a whole lot more in the years to come. We've also examined the role that the first thousand days of life and our childhood can play on our immune health and while this is definitely significant and compelling, it by no means suggests that beyond those years the health of our immune system is out of our control. However, if you are involved in bringing up a child, bearing in mind this information and using it in a way which feels manageable for you can help to set up the child's immune system and health for later on in life.

Clearly we're no longer able to ignore the role of our diet in our overall health and immune system and given the strains on the healthcare system in the UK, it's about time that we take what we can into our own hands to focus more on the prevention of illness rather than the cure. The dietary advice provided in this book can help to nourish your body, your mind and your soul to become a healthier version of yourself. I really hope that you've managed to take away a few key changes which you can begin to implement today. Once you feel you've taken on those changes and they're well integrated into your lifestyle, I urge you to flick back through these pages to find a few more habits that you can begin to implement. Changing your diet and lifestyle to improve your health is a marathon not a sprint. You're far more likely to sustain healthier habits if you incorporate them into your life gradually. It's OK if it takes you years to make changes; you should start to see slow incremental benefits before you reach your final destination and remember, the journey is as important as the destination.

My own fascination with the immune system was born out of my personal experiences but my advice to you is that you definitely shouldn't leave it until there is something to remind you about the importance of the immune system in order to look after it. We can't expect it to look after us in times of need when we're not looking after it on a regular and consistent basis.

The last thought that I'd like to leave you with is to simply remind you about the complexities of the immune system and to highlight that while some products on the market may contribute to supporting a healthier immune function, any which claim to change your life for the better are more often than not far too good to be true. As I've said before, there's no quick fix or magic pill. Improving your health and your immune system requires time, dedication and effort. So please, save your sanity and your money and focus on the core principles of your diet and lifestyle.

Glossary

Adaptive immune system The immune system that adapts over time and learns to respond to specific pathogens

Antioxidants Molecules which donate an extra electron to free radicals in order to stabilise them

B-Lymphocytes (also known as B-cells) Cells that work in collaboration with the T-cells and are able to create a memory of the unwanted pathogens

Basophils These cells are the alarm bells to alert the rest of the immune system that it's under attack

Bioavailability The bioavailability of a nutrient refers to how much of it can be absorbed and utilised in the body

Cell differentiation The process in which cells are provided with their individual specialised roles

Cell proliferation The process in which one cell grows and produces two new cells

Commensal bacteria Beneficial bacterial species which can be found in the gut

Cytokines The messengers of the immune system; they can increase or decrease inflammation

DNA This is the main component of our chromosomes and contains all of our genetic information

Enteropathogens Unwanted pathogens which are carried through soil, food and water

Eosinophils The reserve fighters in the innate immune system

Free radicals Unstable molecules which can contribute to cell damage, cell death and oxidative stress

Gut microbiome Refers to the collection of viruses, bacteria and fungi which are housed within the large intestine

Inflammation A response generated by the immune system in order to alert other immune cells of the targeted site and helps to protect against and fight the attacker. Acute inflammation is short-lived, whereas chronic inflammation is present for a prolonged period of time

Innate immune system The immune system we're born with. It responds in the same manner every time

Leukocytes White blood cells

Lymphocytes These cells attack and kill the unwanted intruders

Metabolic syndrome A term coined for a combination of hypertension, obesity and diabetes

Monocytes These cells break down unwanted bacteria and behave as the cleaning agents to remove destroyed or dead cells

Natural killer cells A type of lymphocyte and a key component of the innate immune system

Neutrophils First responders in the innate immune response

Oxidative stress Occurs as a result of high numbers of free radicals and can contribute to inflammation. A small amount of oxidative stress is considered normal and it can occur through natural processes such as exercise and digestion.

Pathogenic bacteria Negative bacterial species which can be found in the gut

T-lymphocytes (also known as T-cells) The cells responsible for identifying the pathogens and sending messages for help

References

Chapter 2: Introduction to Immunity

Klein, S. L. and Flanagan, K. L., 'Sex differences in immune responses', *Nature Reviews Immunology* 16(10), August 2016, pp. 626–638.

Ghazeeri, G., Abdullah, L., and Abbas, O., 'Immunological differences in women compared with men: overview and contributing factors', *American Journal of Reproductive Immunology* 66(3), September 2011, pp. 163–169.

Bloomfield, S. F., Stanwell Smith, R., Crevel, R. W. R., and Pickup, J., 'Too clean, or not too clean: the hygiene hypothesis and home hygiene', *Clinical & Experimental Allergy* 36(4), April 2006, pp. 402–425.

Crevel, R. and Pickup, M. J., 'The Hygiene Hypothesis and its implications for home hygiene, lifestyle and public health', International Scientific Forum on Home Hygiene, September 2012.

Bloomfield, S. F., 'Is lack of exposure to germs during COVID-19 weakening our immune systems?', International Scientific Forum on Home Hygiene, July 2022.

Scudellari, M., 'Cleaning up the hygiene hypothesis', *Proceedings of the National Academy of Sciences* 114(7), February 2017, pp. 1433–1436.

Chapter 3: The Role of the Gut on Immune Function

Fromm, D., 'How do non-steroidal anti-inflammatory drugs affect gastric mucosal defenses?', *Clinical and Investigative Medicine* 10(3), May 1987, pp. 251–258.

Bishehsari, F., Magno, E., Swanson, G., Desai, V., Voigt, R. M., Forsyth, C. B. and Keshavarzian, A., 'Alcohol and gut-derived inflammation', *Alcohol Research: Current Reviews* 38(2), 2017, p. 163.

Leeuwendaal, N. K., Stanton, C., O'Toole, P. W. and Beresford, T. P, 'Fermented foods, health and the gut microbiome', *Nutrients* 14(7), April 2022, p. 1527.

Hume, M. P., Nicolucci, A. C. and Reimer, R. A., 'Prebiotic supplementation improves appetite control in children with over-weight and obesity: a randomized controlled trial', *American Journal of Clinical Nutrition* 105(4), April 2017, pp. 790–799.

Catalkaya, G., Venema, K., Lucini, L., Rocchetti, G., Delmas, D., Daglia, M. and Capanoglu, E., 'Interaction of dietary polyphenols and gut microbiota: microbial metabolism of polyphenols, influence on the gut microbiota, and implications on host health', *Food Frontiers* 1(2), June 2020, pp. 109–133.

Suez, J., Korem, T., Zeevi, D., Zilberman-Schapira, G., Thaiss, C. A., Maza, O., and Elinav, E., 'Artificial sweeteners induce glucose intolerance by altering the gut microbiota', *Nature* *514*(7521), October 2014, pp. 181–186.

Brookes, Z. L., Belfield, L. A., Ashworth, A., Casas-Agustench, P., Raja, M., Pollard, A. J. and Bescos, R., 'Effects of chlorhexidine mouthwash on the oral microbiome', *Journal of Dentistry 113*, October 2021, p. 103768.

Chapter 4: The Early Years

Robertson, R. C., Manges, A. R., Finlay, B. B. and Prendergast, A. J., 'The human microbiome and child growth – first 1000 days and beyond', *Trends in Microbiology 27*(2), February 2019, pp. 131–147.

Marques, A. H., O'Connor, T. G., Roth, C., Susser, E. and Bjørke-Monsen, A. L., 'The influence of maternal prenatal and early childhood nutrition and maternal prenatal stress on offspring immune system development and neurodevelopmental disorders', *Frontiers in Neuroscience 7*, July 2013, p. 120.

Calder, P. C., 'Feeding the immune system', *Proceedings of the Nutrition Society 72*(3), August 2013, pp. 299–309.

Calder, P. C., Krauss-Etschmann, S., de Jong, E. C., Dupont, C., Frick, J. S., Frokiaer, H., and Koletzko, B., 'Early nutrition and immunity – progress and perspectives', *British Journal of Nutrition 96*(4), October 2006, pp. 774–790.

Ray, C., Kerketta, J. A., Rao, S., Patel, S., Dutt, S., Arora, K., and Bhushan, P., 'Human milk oligosaccharides: The journey ahead', *International Journal of Pediatrics*, August 2019.

Arslanoglu, S., Moro, G. E., Schmitt, J., Tandoi, L., Rizzardi, S. and Boehm, G., 'Early dietary intervention with a mixture of prebiotic oligosaccharides reduces the incidence of allergic manifestations and infections during the first two years of life', *Journal of Nutrition* 138(6), June 2008, pp. 1091–1095.

Fragkou, P. C., Karaviti, D., Zemlin, M. and Skevaki, C., 'Impact of early life nutrition on children's immune system and noncommunicable diseases through its effects on the bacterial microbiome, virome and mycobiome', *Frontiers in Immunology*, March 2021, p. 806.

Food allergies in babies and young children – NHS (https://www.nhs.uk/conditions/baby/weaning-and-feeding/food-allergies-in-babies-and-young-children/).

Chapter 5: The Role of Macronutrients and Micronutrients on Immunity

Spadaro, O., Youm, Y., Shchukina, I., Ryu, S., Sidorov, S., Ravussin, A., and Dixit, V. D, 'Caloric restriction in humans reveals immunometabolic regulators of health span', *Science* 375(6581), February 2022, pp. 671–7.

Li, P., Yin, Y. L., Li, D., Kim, S. W. and Wu, G., 'Amino acids and immune function, *British Journal of Nutrition* 98(2), August 2007, pp. 237–52.

Malaguarnera, L., 'Influence of resveratrol on the immune response', *Nutrients* 11(5), May 2019, p. 946.

Yaqoob, P. and Calder, P. C., 'Fatty acids and immune function:

new insights into mechanisms', *British Journal of Nutrition* *98*(1), October 2007, S41–5.

Gutiérrez, S., Svahn, S. L. and Johansson, M. E., 'Effects of omega-3 fatty acids on immune cells', *International Journal of Molecular Sciences* *20*(20), October 2019, p. 5028.

Hojyo, S. and Fukada, T, 'Roles of zinc signaling in the immune system', *Journal of Immunology Research*, 2016.

Yates, C. M., Calder, P. C. and Rainger, G. E., 'Pharmacology and therapeutics of omega-3 polyunsaturated fatty acids in chronic inflammatory disease', *Pharmacology & Therapeutics* *141*(3), March 2014, pp. 272–82.

Calder, P. C., 'Fatty acids and inflammation: the cutting edge between food and pharma', *European Journal of Pharmacology* *668*, September 2011, S50–8.

Chishaki, T., Umeda, T., Takahashi, I., Matsuzaka, M., Iwane, K., Matsumoto, H., and Nakaji, S., 'Effects of dehydration on immune functions after a judo practice session', *Luminescence* *28*(2), March–April 2013, pp. 114–120.

Gombart, A. F., Pierre, A. and Maggini, S., 'A review of micronutrients and the immune system – working in harmony to reduce the risk of infection', *Nutrients* *12*(1), January 2020, p. 236.

Qian, B., Shen, S., Zhang, J. and Jing, P., 'Effects of vitamin B6 deficiency on the composition and functional potential of T cell populations', *Journal of Immunology Research*, 2017.

Mikkelsen, K. and Apostolopoulos, V., 'Vitamin B12, folic acid, and the immune system', *Nutrition and Immunity*, July 2019, pp. 103–114.

Carr, A. C. and Maggini, S., 'Vitamin C and immune function', *Nutrients* 9(11), November 2017, p. 1211.

NDNS: results from years 9 to 11 (combined) statistical summary – GOV.UK (https://www.gov.uk/government/statistics/ndns-results-from-years-9-to-11-2016-to-2017-and-2018-to-2019/ndns-results-from-years-9-to-11-combined-statistical-summary).

Chapter 6: Incorporating Immune-friendly Foods Into Your Diet

Salman H., Bergman, M., Djaldetti, M., Orlin, J. and Bessler, H., 'Citrus pectin affects cytokine production by human peripheral blood mononuclear cells', *Biomedicine & Pharmacotherapy* 62(9), November 2008, pp. 579–82.

Hosseini, B., Berthon, B. S., Saedisomeolia, A., Starkey, M. R., Collison, A., Wark, P. A. and Wood, L. G., 'Effects of fruit and vegetable consumption on inflammatory biomarkers and immune cell populations: a systematic literature review and meta-analysis', *American Journal of Clinical Nutrition*, 108(1), 2018, pp. 136–155.

Gibson, A., Edgar, J. D., Neville, C. E., Gilchrist, S. E., McKinley, M. C., Patterson, C. C. and Woodside, J. V., 'Effect of fruit and vegetable consumption on immune function in older people: a randomized controlled trial', *American Journal of Clinical Nutrition* 96(6), December 2012, pp. 1429–36. Kadyan, S., Sharma, A., Arjmandi, B. H., Singh, P. and Nagpal, R., 'Prebiotic potential of dietary beans and pulses and their resistant starch for aging-associated gut and metabolic health', *Nutrients* 14(9), April 2022, p. 1726.

De, L. C., 'Edible seeds and nuts in human diet for immunity development', *International Journal of Recent Science Research* 6(11), June 2020, pp. 38877–81.

Vanegas, S. M., Meydani, M., Barnett, J. B., Goldin, B., Kane, A., Rasmussen, H. and Meydani, S. N., 'Substituting whole grains for refined grains in a 6-wk randomized trial has a modest effect on gut microbiota and immune and inflammatory markers of healthy adults', *American Journal of Clinical Nutrition* 105(3), March 2017, pp. 635–50.

Kim, J. E. and Campbell, W. W., 'Dietary cholesterol contained in whole eggs is not well absorbed and does not acutely affect plasma total cholesterol concentration in men and women: results from 2 randomized controlled crossover studies', *Nutrients* 10(9), September 2018, p. 1272.

Blesso, C. N. and Fernandez, M. L., 'Dietary cholesterol, serum lipids, and heart disease: are eggs working for or against you?', *Nutrients* 10(4), March 2018, p. 426.

Guldiken, B., Ozkan, G., Catalkaya, G., Ceylan, F. D., Yalcinkaya, I. E. and Capanoglu, E., 'Phytochemicals of herbs and spices: Health versus toxicological effects', *Food and Chemical Toxicology 119*, September 2018, pp. 37–49. Vafaeipour, Z., Razavi, B. M. and Hosseinzadeh, H., 'Effects of turmeric (Curcuma longa) and its constituent (curcumin) on the metabolic syndrome: an updated review', *Journal of Integrative Medicine* 20(3), May 2022, pp. 193–203.

Razavi, B. M., Ghasemzadeh Rahbardar, M. and Hosseinzadeh, H., 'A review of therapeutic potentials of turmeric (Curcuma longa) and its active constituent, curcumin, on inflammatory disorders, pain, and their related patents', *Phytotherapy Research* 35(12), December 2021, pp. 6489–6513.

Ballester, P., Cerdá, B., Arcusa, R., Marhuenda, J., Yamedjeu, K. and Zafrilla, P., 'Effect of Ginger on Inflammatory Diseases', *Molecules* 27(21), November 2022, p. 7223.

Arreola, R., Quintero-Fabián, S., López-Roa, R. I., Flores-Gutiérrez, E. O., Reyes-Grajeda, J. P., Carrera-Quintanar, L. and Ortuño-Sahagún, D., 'Immunomodulation and anti-inflammatory effects of garlic compounds', *Journal of Immunology Research*, April 2015.

Londhe, V. P., Gavasane, A. T., Nipate, S. S., Bandawane, D. D. and Chaudhari, P. D., 'Role of garlic (Allium sativum) in various diseases: an overview', *Angiogenesis* 12(13), January 2011, pp. 129–34.

Popa, M. E., Mitelut, A. C., Popa, E. E., Stan, A. and Popa, V. I., 'Organic foods contribution to nutritional quality and value', *Trends in Food Science & Technology 84*, February 2019, pp. 15–18.

Błaszczyk, N., Rosiak, A. and Kałuna-Czapliska, J., 'The potential role of cinnamon in human health', *Forests 12*(5), May 2021, p. 648. Hariri, M. and Ghiasvand, R., 'Cinnamon and chronic diseases', *Drug Discovery from Mother Nature*, 2016, pp. 1–24.

Chapter 7: Dietary Components Hindering Our Immunity

Shomali, N., Mahmoudi, J., Mahmoodpoor, A., Zamiri, R. E., Akbari, M., Xu, H. and Shotorbani, S. S., 'Harmful effects of high amounts of glucose on the immune system: an updated review', *Biotechnology and Applied Biochemistry 68*(2), April 2021, pp. 404–410.

Jafar, N., Edriss, H. and Nugent, K., 'The effect of short-term hyperglycemia on the innate immune system', *American Journal of the Medical Sciences 351*(2), February 2016, pp. 201–211.

Clement, C. C., Nanaware, P. P., Yamazaki, T., Negroni, M. P., Ramesh, K., Morozova, K., and Santambrogio, L., 'Pleiotropic consequences of metabolic stress for the major histocompatibility complex class II molecule antigen processing and presentation machinery', *Immunity 54*(4), April 2021, pp. 721–36.

Santos, H. O., de Moraes, W. M., da Silva, G. A., Prestes, J. and Schoenfeld, B. J., 'Vinegar (acetic acid) intake on glucose metabolism: a narrative review', *Clinical Nutrition ESPEN 32*, August 2019, pp. 1–7. Shishehbor, F., Mansoori, A. and Shirani, F., 'Vinegar consumption can attenuate postprandial glucose and insulin responses; a systematic review and meta-analysis of clinical trials', *Diabetes Research and Clinical Practice 127*, May 2017, pp. 1–9.

Zani, F., Blagih, J., Gruber, T., Buck, M. D., Jones, N., Hennequart, M., and Vousden, K. H., 'The dietary sweetener sucralose is a negative modulator of T cell-mediated responses', *Nature*, March 2023, pp. 1–7.

Basson, A. R., Rodriguez-Palacios, A. and Cominelli, F., 'Artificial sweeteners: history and new concepts on inflammation', *Frontiers in Nutrition 8*, September 2021, 746247. Suez, J., Korem, T., Zeevi, D., Zilberman-Schapira, G., Thaiss, C. A., Maza, O., and Elinav, E., 'Artificial sweeteners induce glucose intolerance by altering the gut microbiota', *Nature* 514(7521), October 2014, pp. 181–6.

Paula Neto, H. A., Ausina, P., Gomez, L. S., Leandro, J. G., Zancan, P. and Sola-Penna, M., 'Effects of food additives on immune cells as contributors to body weight gain and immune-mediated metabolic dysregulation', *Frontiers in Immunology 8*, November 2017, p. 1478.

Bischoff, N. S., de Kok, T. M., Sijm, D. T., van Breda, S. G., Briedé, J. J., Castenmiller, J. J., and Van Loveren, H., 'Possible adverse effects of food additive E171 (titanium dioxide) related to particle specific human toxicity, including the immune system', *International Journal of Molecular Sciences 22*(1), December 2020, p. 207.

Banerjee, A., Mukherjee, S. and Maji, B. K., 'Worldwide flavor enhancer monosodium glutamate combined with high lipid diet provokes metabolic alterations and systemic anom-alies: an overview', *Toxicology Reports 8*, 2021, pp. 938–61. National Diet and Nutrition Survey: Assessment of salt intake from urinary sodium in adults (publishing.service.gov. uk) (page 23)

Willebrand, R. and Kleinewietfeld, M., 'The role of salt for immune cell function and disease', *Immunology 154*(3), July 2018, pp. 346–53.

Yi, B., Titze, J., Rykova, M., Feuerecker, M., Vassilieva, G., Nichiporuk, I. and Choukèr, A., 'Effects of dietary salt levels on monocytic cells and immune responses in healthy human subjects: a longitudinal study', *Translational Research 166*(1), July 2015, pp. 103–110.

NDNS: results from years 9 to 11 (combined) – statistical summary, GOV.UK (https://www.gov.uk/government/statistics/ndns-results-from-years-9-to-11-2016-to-2017-and-2018-to-2019/ndns-results-from-years-9-to-11-combined-statistical-summary)

Schwartz, E. A., Zhang, W. Y., Karnik, S. K., Borwege, S., Anand, V. R., Laine, P. S. and Reaven, P. D., 'Nutrient modification of the innate immune response: a novel mechanism by which saturated fatty acids greatly amplify monocyte inflammation', *Arteriosclerosis, Thrombosis, and Vascular Biology 30*(4), April 2010, pp. 802–8.

Chapter 8: Autoimmunity and Dietary Patterns Associated with Autoimmune Conditions

Mazzucca, C. B., Raineri, D., Cappellano, G. and Chiocchetti, A., 'How to tackle the relationship between autoimmune diseases and diet: well begun is half-done', *Nutrients 13*(11), November 2021, p. 3956.

Manzel, A., Muller, D. N., Hafler, D. A., Erdman, S. E., Linker, R. A. and Kleinewietfeld, M., 'Role of "Western diet" in inflammatory autoimmune diseases', *Current Allergy and Asthma Reports 14*, January 2014, pp.1–8.

Christ, A., Lauterbach, M. and Latz, E., 'Western diet and the immune system: an inflammatory connection', *Immunity 51*(5), November 2019, pp. 794–811.

Statovci, D., Aguilera, M., MacSharry, J. and Melgar, S., 'The impact of western diet and nutrients on the microbiota and immune response at mucosal interfaces', *Frontiers in Immunology 8*, July 2017, p. 838.

Casas, R., Sacanella, E. and Estruch, R., 'The immune protective effect of the Mediterranean diet against chronic low-grade inflammatory diseases', *Endocrine, Metabolic & Immune Disorders-Drug Targets* 14(4), 2014, pp. 245–54.

Tsigalou, C., Tsolou, A., Konstantinidis, T., Zafiriou, E., Efthimios, D., Tsirogianni, A. and Bogdanos, D., 'Interplay between Mediterranean diet and gut microbiota in the interface of auto-immunity: an overview', *Preprints.org*, 2020, pp. 8–10.

Martínez-González, M. A., Salas-Salvadó, J., Estruch, R., Corella, D., Fitó, M., Ros, E., and Predimed Investigators (2015), 'Benefits of the Mediterranean diet: insights from the PREDIMED study', *Progress in Cardiovascular Diseases*, 58(1), 50–60.

Picchianti Diamanti, A., Panebianco, C., Salerno, G., Di Rosa, R., Salemi, S., Sorgi, M. L., and Laganà, B., 'Impact of Mediterranean diet on disease activity and gut microbiota composition of rheumatoid arthritis patients', *Microorganisms* 8(12), December 2020, p. 1989.

Bolla, A. M., Caretto, A., Laurenzi, A., Scavini, M. and Piemonti, L., 'Low-carb and ketogenic diets in type 1 and type 2 diabetes', *Nutrients* 11(5), May 2019, p. 962.

Zhu, H., Bi, D., Zhang, Y., Kong, C., Du, J., Wu, X. and Qin, H., 'Ketogenic diet for human diseases: the underlying mechanisms and potential for clinical implementations', *Signal Transduction and Targeted Therapy* 7(1), January 2022, p. 11.

Chapter 9: Lifestyle Factors Affecting Immune Function

Cohen, S., Doyle, W. J., Alper, C. M., Janicki-Deverts, D. and Turner, R. B., 'Sleep habits and susceptibility to the common cold', *Archives of Internal Medicine* 169(1), January 2009, pp. 62–7. Motivala, S. J. and Irwin, M. R., 'Sleep and immunity: cytokine pathways linking sleep and health outcomes', *Current Directions in Psychological Science* 16(1), 2007, pp. 21–5.

de Almeida, C. M. O. and Malheiro, A., 'Sleep, immunity and shift workers: A review', *Sleep Science* 9(3), July–September 2016, pp. 164–8.

Zimmermann, P. and Curtis, N., 'Factors that influence the immune response to vaccination', *Clinical Microbiology Reviews* 32(2), March 2019, e00084–18.

Spiegel, K., Tasali, E., Leproult, R., and Van Cauter, E. (2009), 'Effects of poor and short sleep on glucose metabolism and obesity risk', *Nature Reviews Endocrinology*, 5(5), pp. 253–261.

Rodak, K., Kokot, I. and Kratz, E. M., 'Caffeine as a factor influencing the functioning of the human body – Friend or foe?', *Nutrients* 13(9), September 2021, p. 3088.

Statistics on Alcohol, England 2021 – NHS Digital (https://digital.nhs.uk/data-and-information/publications/statistical/statistics-on-alcohol/2021).

Sarkar, D., Jung, M. K. and Wang, H. J., 'Alcohol and the immune system', *Alcohol Research: Current Reviews* 37(2), 2015, p. 153.

Adult smoking habits in the UK – Office for National Statistics (https://www.ons.gov.uk/peoplepopulationandcommunity/healthandsocialcare/healthandlifeexpectancies/bulletins/adultsmokinghabitsingreatbritain/2019).

Alrouji, M., Manouchehrinia, A., Gran, B. and Constantinescu, C. S., 'Effects of cigarette smoke on immunity, neuroinflammation and multiple sclerosis', *Journal of Neuroimmunology 329*, April 2019, pp. 24–34.

Qiu, F., Liang, C. L., Liu, H., Zeng, Y. Q., Hou, S., Huang, S. and Dai, Z., 'Impacts of cigarette smoking on immune responsiveness: up and down or upside down?', *Oncotarget 8*(1), January 2017, p. 268.

Costenbader, K. H. and Karlson, E. W., 'Cigarette smoking and autoimmune disease: what can we learn from epidemiology?', *Lupus 15*(11), 2006, pp. 737–745.

Dhabhar, F. S., 'Effects of stress on immune function: the good, the bad, and the beautiful', *Immunologic Research 58*, May 2014, pp. 193–210.

Bae, Y. S., Shin, E. C., Bae, Y. S. and Van Eden, W., 'Stress and immunity', *Frontiers in Immunology 10*, February 2019, p. 245.

Black, D. S. and Slavich, G. M., 'Mindfulness meditation and the immune system: a systematic review of randomized controlled trials', *Annals of the New York Academy of Sciences 1373*(1), June 2016, pp. 13–24. Laddu, D. R., Lavie, C. J., Phillips, S. A. and Arena, R., 'Physical activity for immunity protection: inoculating populations with healthy living medicine in preparation for the next pandemic', *Progress in Cardiovascular Diseases 64*, January–February 2021, p. 102.

Nieman, D. C., Henson, D. A., Austin, M. D. and Sha, W., 'Upper respiratory tract infection is reduced in physically fit and active adults', *British Journal of Sports Medicine* 45(12), September 2011, pp. 987–92. Cerdá, B., Pérez, M., Pérez-Santiago, J. D., Tornero-Aguilera, J. F., González-Soltero, R. and Larrosa, M., 'Gut microbiota modification: another piece in the puzzle of the benefits of physical exercise in health?', *Frontiers in Physiology* 7, February 2016, p. 51.

Barton, W., Penney, N. C., Cronin, O., Garcia-Perez, I., Molloy, M. G., Holmes, E. and O'Sullivan, O. (2018), 'The microbiome of professional athletes differs from that of more sedentary subjects in composition and particularly at the functional metabolic level', *Gut*, 67(4), pp. 625–633. Wegierska, A. E., Charitos, I. A., Topi, S., Potenza, M. A., Montagnani, M. and Santacroce, L., 'The connection between physical exercise and gut microbiota: implications for competitive sports athletes', *Sports Medicine* 52(10), May 2022, pp. 2355–69. Simpson, R. J., Campbell, J. P., Gleeson, M., Krüger, K., Nieman, D. C., Pyne, D. B. and Walsh, N. P., 'Can exercise affect immune function to increase susceptibility to infection?', *Exercise Immunology Review* 26, 2020, pp. 8–22. Spence, L., Brown, W. J., Pyne, D. B., Nissen, M. D., Sloots, T. P., McCormack, J. G. and Fricker, P. A., 'Incidence, etiology, and symptomatology of upper respiratory illness in elite athletes', *Medicine & Science in Sports & Exercise* 39(4), April 2007, pp. 577–86. Bresnahan, R., 'Cold water immersion and anti-inflammatory response: A systematic review', *Exercise & Sport Nutrition Reviews*, August 2019.

Goedsche, K., Förster, M., Kroegel, C. and Uhlemann, C., 'Repeated cold water stimulations (hydrotherapy according to Kneipp) in patients with COPD', *Forschende Komplementarmedizin* 14(3), June 2007, pp. 158–66.

Tipton, M., Massey, H., Mayhew, A. and Morgan, P., 'Cold water therapies: minimising risks', *British Journal of Sports Medicine* 56(23), September 2022, pp. 1332–34.

Ural, B. B. and Farber, D. L., 'Effect of air pollution on the human immune system', *Nature Medicine 28*, November 2022, pp. 2622–32.

Orysiak, J., Młynarczyk, M., Piec, R. and Jakubiak, A., 'Lifestyle and environmental factors may induce airway and systemic inflammation in firefighters', *Environmental Science and Pollution Research 29*(49), October 2022, pp. 73741–68.

Gameiro, C. M., Romão, F. and Castelo-Branco, C., 'Menopause and aging: changes in the immune system – a review', *Maturitas*, 67(4), December 2010, pp. 316–20.

Romao, F. and Gameiro, C., 'Changes in the immune system during menopause and aging', *Frontiers in Bioscience-Elite* 2(4), June 2010, pp. 1299–1303.

Min, J., Jo, H., Chung, Y. J., Song, J. Y., Kim, M. J. and Kim, M. R., 'Vitamin D and the immune system in menopause: a review', *Journal of Menopausal Medicine 27*(3), December 2021, p. 109.

Hannan, M. A., Rahman, M. A., Rahman, M. S., Sohag, A. A. M., Dash, R., Hossain, K. S. and Uddin, M. J. 'Intermittent fasting, a possible priming tool for host defense against SARS-CoV-2 infection: crosstalk among calorie restriction, autophagy and immune response', *Immunology Letters 226*, October 2020, pp. 38–45.

Cui, B., Lin, H., Yu, J., Yu, J. and Hu, Z., 'Autophagy and the immune response', *Autophagy: Biology and Diseases: Basic Science*, September 2019, pp. 595–634.

Ownby, D. R., Johnson, C. C. and Peterson, E. L., 'Exposure to dogs and cats in the first year of life and risk of allergic sensitization at 6 to 7 years of age', *JAMA*, *288*(8), August 2022, pp. 963–72.

Nafstad, P., Magnus, P., Gaarder, P. I. and Jaakkola, J. J. K., 'Exposure to pets and atopy-related diseases in the first 4 years of life', *Allergy 56*(4), April 2011, pp. 307–12.

Chapter 10: Should I Be Taking Supplements?

Calder, P. C., Carr, A. C., Gombart, A. F. and Eggersdorfer, M., 'Optimal nutritional status for a well-functioning immune system is an important factor to protect against viral infections', *Nutrients 12*(4), April 2020, p. 1181.

Hemilä, H., 'Vitamin C and infections', *Nutrients 9*(4), April 2017, p. 339.

Hemilä, H. and Chalker, E., 'Vitamin C for preventing and treating the common cold', *Cochrane Database of Systematic Reviews* (1), January 2013.

DiNicolantonio, J. J. and O'Keefe, J. H., 'Magnesium and vitamin D deficiency as a potential cause of immune dysfunction, cytokine storm and disseminated intravascular coagulation in COVID-19 patients', *Missouri Medicine 118*(1), January–February 2021, p. 68.

Prietl, B., Treiber, G., Pieber, T. R. and Amrein, K., 'Vitamin D and immune function', *Nutrients* 5(7), July 2013, pp. 2502–21. Cannell, J. J., Vieth, R., Umhau, J. C., Holick, M. F., Grant, W. B., Madronich, S. and Giovannucci, E., 'Epidemic influenza and vitamin D', *Epidemiology & Infection* 134(6), December 2006, pp. 1129–40.

Hornsby, E., Pfeffer, P. E., Laranjo, N., Cruikshank, W., Tuzova, M., Litonjua, A. A. and Hawrylowicz, C., 'Vitamin D supplementation during pregnancy: effect on the neonatal immune system in a randomized controlled trial', *Journal of Allergy and Clinical Immunology* 141(1), January 2018, pp. 269–78. Maier, J. A., Castiglioni, S., Locatelli, L., Zocchi, M. and Mazur, A., 'Magnesium and inflammation: Advances and perspectives', *Seminars in Cell & Developmental Biology* 115, July 2021, pp. 37–44. Chasapis, C. T., Ntoupa, P. S. A., Spiliopoulou, C. A. and Stefanidou, M. E., 'Recent aspects of the effects of zinc on human health', *Archives of Toxicology* 94, May 2020, pp. 1443–60.

Bonaventura, P., Benedetti, G., Albarède, F. and Miossec, P., 'Zinc and its role in immunity and inflammation', *Autoimmunity Reviews* 14(4), April 2015, pp. 277–85.

Galdeano, C. M., Cazorla, S. I., Dumit, J. M. L., Vélez, E. and Perdigón, G., 'Beneficial effects of probiotic consumption on the immune system', *Annals of Nutrition and Metabolism* 74(2), 2019, pp. 115–24.

Yan, F. and Polk, D. B., 'Probiotics and immune health', *Current Opinion in Gastroenterology* 27(6), October 2011, p. 496.

Index

Note: page numbers in *italics* refer to information contained in tables. Recipe titles are grouped under the index heading 'recipes'.

Acknowledgements

This book has been a labour of love and an opportunity for which I'm forever grateful. I couldn't have written it without the support of an incredible team.

To my family:

My husband Adrian, thank you for supporting me and pushing me in ways I didn't know I could be pushed. Thank you for always showing up and encouraging me through everything I do. I really would be lost without you.

To my parents and my brother, thank you for teaching me a good work ethic from day one, for always encouraging me to step outside my comfort zone and for being the most incredible support system I could have ever asked for. You are truly special people and I'm forever grateful for having you in my life. Dad, thank you for always having the answer to any problem and for teaching me all your life experience. Mum, thank you for being such an inspiration, for standing by my side throughout my life and for encouraging me to explore the world of nutrition.

To my extended family and my friends who are like family, thank you for your endless support and positivity. Thank you for fuelling my social wellbeing, for always being there to share some delicious food, a good natter or a few glasses of wine. You do more for my social and mental wellbeing than you'll ever know.

To my agents at Northbank Talent, Matthew and Diane, thank you for all your support, guidance, help and advice on making this book become a reality.

To the team at Piatkus, Zoe, Jillian, Clare and Narjas, thank you for believing in me and trusting me to write this book. I truly appreciate being able to work with such a wonderful and talented team who share the same approach and vision for this book. You've been an absolute pleasure to work with and for that I am incredibly grateful.

And to you, the reader, thank you for purchasing this book, for your support and for trusting me to share this knowledge and advice with you. I really hope this book can help you to make healthier changes and improve your general wellbeing.